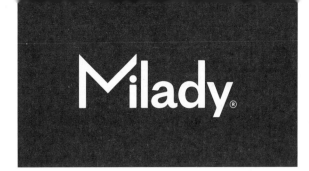

Advanced Services

Eyelashes

Eyelash Extensions

1st EDITION

www.milady.com

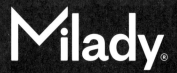

Advanced Services

Eyelashes

1st EDITION

Senior Vice President and General Manager: Sandra Bruce

Vice President, Milady Product & Customer Experience: Corina Santoro

Associate Product Manager: Sarah Koumourdas

Content Creation Manager: Jessica Mahoney

Senior Content Manager: Nina Tucciarelli

Content Manager: Kelsy Nevins

Digital Content Manager: Kim Morté

Content Project Manager: Michael Dee

Product Assistant: Amanda Conley-Killian

Manager, Digital Production and Customer Support: Danielle Hannigan

Digital Content Specialists: Jean Choe and Christine Stavrou

Senior Marketing Director: Slavik Volinsky

Senior Marketing Manager: Kim Berube

In-House Subject Matter Expert: Harry Garrott

Associate Creative Director: Wood Dabbs

Production Service: MPS Limited

Cover Image Source: Mama Bear LA

Copyright © 2023 Cengage Learning, Inc. ALL RIGHTS RESERVED.

No part of this work covered by the copyright herein may be reproduced or distributed in any form or by any means, except as permitted by U.S. copyright law, without the prior written permission of the copyright owner.

Unless otherwise noted, all content is Copyright © Cengage Learning, Inc.

For Milady product information, visit **milady.com**
For technical assistance or support, visit **milady.com/help**

For permission to use material from this text or product, submit all requests online at **www.copyright.com**.

Library of Congress Control Number: 2022917291

ISBN: 978-0-357-92320-7

Milady, a part of Cengage Group
200 Pier 4 Boulevard
Boston, MA 02210
USA

Milady hasn't just set the standard for beauty education. We continually raise it with every product and feature release to meet the needs of today's learners, educators, and employers. Get the full story at **milady.com/about**.

Notice to the Reader
Publisher does not warrant or guarantee any of the products described herein or perform any independent analysis in connection with any of the product information contained herein. Publisher does not assume, and expressly disclaims, any obligation to obtain and include information other than that provided to it by the manufacturer. The reader is expressly warned to consider and adopt all safety precautions that might be indicated by the activities described herein and to avoid all potential hazards. By following the instructions contained herein, the reader willingly assumes all risks in connection with such instructions. The publisher makes no representations or warranties of any kind, including but not limited to, the warranties of fitness for particular purpose or merchantability, nor are any such representations implied with respect to the material set forth herein, and the publisher takes no responsibility with respect to such material. The publisher shall not be liable for any special, consequential, or exemplary damages resulting, in whole or part, from the readers' use of, or reliance upon, this material.

Printed in the United States of America.

Print Number: 02   Print Year: 2022

Brief Contents

01	Chapter 01 **Eyelash Extension History and Careers**	p. 002
02	Chapter 02 **Eye and Eyelash Anatomy and Physiology**	p. 016
03	Chapter 03 **Disorders, Diseases, and Allergies of the Eye Area**	p. 034
04	Chapter 04 **Client Safety and Infection Control**	p. 048
05	Chapter 05 **Tools, Products, and Ingredients**	p. 084
06	Chapter 06 **Eyelash Extension Application**	p. 110
07	Chapter 07 **Eyelash and Eyebrow Chemical Services**	p. 164
08	Chapter 08 **Building an Eyelash Business**	p. 198
References		p. 220
Glossary		p. 222
Index		p. 228

Contents

Chapter 01 | 002

Eyelash Extension History and Careers

- 004 Why Study Eyelash Extension History and Careers?
- 005 History of Eyelash Enhancements
- 009 Scope of Practice and Laws
- 012 Overview of the Eyelash Industry

Chapter 02 | 016

Eye and Eyelash Anatomy and Physiology

- 018 Why Study Anatomy and Physiology of the Eye?
- 019 Anatomy of the Eye
- 023 Eye and Eyelid Shapes
- 025 Eye Spacing on the Face
- 030 Eyelash Hair Growth Stages

Chapter 03 | 034

Disorders, Diseases, and Allergies of the Eye Area

- 036 Why Study Disorders, Diseases, and Allergies of the Eye Area?
- 037 Disorders and Diseases of the Eye Area
- 042 Allergy Versus Sensitivity

Chapter 04 | 048

Client Safety and Infection Control

- 050 Why Study Client Safety and Infection Control?
- 051 Infection Control Basics
- 053 Hand Washing
- 056 Cleaning and Disinfecting
- 064 Exposure Incidents

Chapter 05 | 084

Tools, Products, and Ingredients

- 086 Why Study Tools, Products, and Ingredients?
- 087 Adhesives
- 092 Implements, Tools, and Equipment
- 099 Eyelash Extensions
- 103 Service Products and Ingredients

Chapter 06 | 110
Eyelash Extension Application

- 112 Why Study Eyelash Extension Application?
- 113 Client Consultation
- 117 Choosing the Proper Extension
- 120 Eyelash Mapping
- 124 Contraindications
- 126 Preparation for Extensions
- 130 Temporary Eyelash Application
- 132 Classic Eyelash Application
- 135 Volume Eyelash Application
- 137 Eyelash Refill
- 140 Eyelash Extension Removal
- 142 Client Aftercare
- 144 Troubleshooting

Chapter 07 | 164
Eyelash and Eyebrow Chemical Services

- 166 Why Study Eyelash and Eyebrow Chemical Services?
- 167 Client Consultation
- 170 Client Aftercare
- 172 Eyelash Lifting (Perming)
- 176 Eyebrow Lamination
- 179 Eyelash Tinting
- 182 Eyebrow Tinting

Chapter 08 | 198
Building an Eyelash Business

- 200 Why Study How to Build an Eyelash Business?
- 201 Professional Image
- 204 Ethics
- 207 Choosing Products
- 209 Pricing Services
- 211 Retailing
- 212 Marketing
- 217 Social Media

Procedures

4-1	Proper Hand Washing	069
4-2	Cleaning and Disinfecting Nonporous, Reusable Items	071
4-3	Pre-Service Procedure	073
4-4	Post-Service Procedure	077
4-5	Handling an Exposure Incident: Client Injury	080
4-6	Handling an Exposure Incident: Employee Injury	082
6-1	Temporary Eyelash Strip Application	148
6-2	Temporary Eyelash Cluster Application	150
6-3	Classic Eyelash Application	153
6-4	Volume Eyelash Application	156
6-5	Eyelash Refill	159
6-6	Eyelash Extension Removal	161
7-1	Eyelash Lifting (Perming)	185
7-2	Eyebrow Lamination	189
7-3	Eyelash Tinting	192
7-4	Eyebrow Tinting	195

Preface

It Starts with a Passion and Becomes a Thriving Career

You've made the right choice. Whether you're seeking a career in esthetics, cosmetology, or simply want to specialize in eyelash services you're redefining success by pursuing the work you love while making a difference in people's lives. That's huge, so don't let anybody say otherwise.

We proudly own our craft and are here to prove that a career in beauty and wellness can lead to professional success and personal fulfillment. We see it happen all the time, and we have full confidence that by putting in the work, getting your hands dirty, and taking risks, you'll reach your dreams: whatever they look like. And together with your educators, Milady is here to support you every step of the way.

Welcome to the industry where your passion will become a thriving career.

Let's Push the Beauty Industry Forward

At Milady, we believe that careers in beauty are legitimate paths to success with the potential to make a difference. How do we know? Simple: It's in our history.

Milady has been influencing the beauty industry for nearly a century—starting with our founder Nick Cimaglia, an Italian immigrant who launched a one-man barbering supply business. Our beginnings were humble, but they were also visionary—a vision that continues to guide us today.

For our students, this means giving you a modern digital platform, up-to-date content, detailed step-by-step instructions, engaging visuals and videos, and inspiring concepts that are applicable no matter what product line your school or future spa/salon carries . . . and no matter how big your dreams are.

I welcome you to this exciting industry—an industry where we're redefining what it means to be a beauty professional and expanding the possibilities of what beauty can do for an individual, a community, and the world. I'm thrilled to have you join us and can't wait to see what you do next.

Are you ready to put in the work, get your hands dirty, and take (smart) risks? Of course you are. That's why you're here. Sign your name below and take the pledge.

I am willing to put in the work, get my hands dirty, and take smart risks to reach professional success and personal fulfillment:

Name   Date

Sandra Bruce
SVP and General Manager, Milady

How to Use this Text

In response to advances in learning science and the growing importance of competency-based education, several features have been added with the hope of making your learning experience more intuitive, more effective, and above all more relevant.

Learning Objectives

At the beginning of every chapter is a list of learning objectives that tells you what important information you will be expected to know after studying the chapter. These learning objectives are attached to the major sections of each chapter for ease of reference and to reinforce the main competencies that are critical to learn for course completion and/or certification. In addition, learning objectives have been written to focus on measurable results, helping you know what it is you should be able to do after mastering each section.

Check In Questions

Instead of placing review questions at the end of each chapter, Check In questions have been added to the end of the relevant section. This allows you to check your understanding as you progress through a chapter, as opposed to waiting until you have finished the chapter to check your memory. Check In questions also make it easier to find any answers you need help with.

Workbook Assessments

At the end of each section are assessments that you might be used to finding in a separate workbook. These assessments test your comprehension of that section's content and are useful for added review before the chapter exam. Assessments may take the form of case study (multiple choice), fill in the blank, matching, multiple response (choose all that apply), true or false, and more.

Meet the Contributors

Milady recognizes the many gifts and talents of its contributors worldwide. It is with gratitude that we thank these very special contributors of the 1st edition of *Milady Advanced Services: Eyelashes*! Every contributor is a unique educational resource whose experiences and achievements continue to expand over time. We are pleased to share their current biographies and a glimpse into what they have accomplished below.

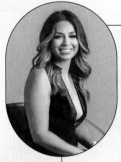

GABRIELA "GABY" CHAVEZ

"Set goals so big they laugh, then cry as they watch you succeed."

Gabriela Chavez has been in the eyelash industry for over 10 years and is currently the proud owner of Learn.LASH.Repeat Training Academy in Dallas, TX. She is one of Dallas's top recognized lash educators, with multiple lash extension and lift certificates from all across the United States. Gabys' driving goal is to improve the quality and standards set in the lash industry. She believes all students, old and new alike, deserve in-depth training and high-quality supplies to ensure lash artists have the skills, knowledge, and support to continually thrive as entrepreneurs in the lash industry. We can learn so much from one another while maintaining our own unique techniques.

CORTNEY LEDUC

Cutting her dolls' hair and braiding all her teammates' is how Cortney Leduc discovered her passion for the cosmetology industry. Over 15 years of experience later, and with a little extra kick, she found herself wanting something more challenging in life.

From working behind the chair as a hair artist, making guests feel incredible, and listening to their life experiences, Cortney knew she wanted to go further and help build future salon leaders. When the opportunity arose, she and her business partner, Julie, came together and opened The Salon Professional Academy, an award-winning cosmetology school in Maplewood, MN. Cortney continues to expand her personal education in all facets of cosmetology, by training in the latest hair trends, business strategies, and leadership skills.

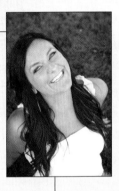

Meet the Contributors

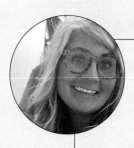

JORDAN MAHRER

Jordan Mahrer is a wife, mother, stylist, lash artist, and lead educator at an award-winning cosmetology school in Maplewood, MN. Her introduction to the industry began in the days of coloring her own hair in the bathroom, getting into her mom's colored eyeliners, and having a daughter with the most unruly curly hair. It truly flourished when she enrolled at the Regency Beauty Institute in the summer of 2014. During her time in cosmetology school, she was an active member on student council, achieved both designer and master designer status, and obtained a salon job prior to graduating in 2015. While working full time in the salon, Jordan continued her education, taking many classes and achieving multiple certifications. Some of the things she is most proud of being certified in are Brazilian blowouts, eyelash extensions, multiple brands of hair extensions, as well as safety and sanitation. Education is Jordan's biggest passion, so it is no surprise that in 2019 she received her cosmetology instructor's license. Jordan's dedication and determination have provided many opportunities for growth and fueled her ability to give back to future industry professionals.

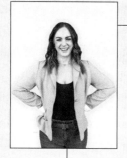

AMANDA JEAN MESSERLI

Amanda Jean Messerli is an esthetician with 15 years in the beauty industry under her belt. She dove into lash extensions 8 years ago and has never looked back! While attending the Aveda Institute in Seattle, WA, Amanda fell in love with all things beauty. She is seven times certified in lashes, specializing in Russian Volume application. Amanda currently has two thriving lash studios in Reno, NV— Midtown Beauty Bar and Midtown Beauty Bar II—with no plans to stop any time soon. Driven by her passion for the industry, Amanda is now teaching others how to build a successful lash business and empower themselves through education.

Meet the Contributors

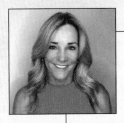

ANNE MILLER

Anne Miller is a master lash artist, an educator, and the founder of E'lan Lashes Eyelash Extensions. She began her career as an entrepreneur in the beauty industry 21 years ago, finding her passion for lashes in 2006. As a visionary and industry leader, Anne is one of the pioneers of eyelash extension certification training in the United States. Through continued research and education, she has made it her mission to bring the finest products and lash certification training to educators across the country. E'lan Lashes has been featured in several major trade publications such as *American Spa*, *Beauty Store Business*, *Update*, and *Modern Salon*, to name a few.

Anne has trained thousands of lash artists and cosmetology school educators over the past 16 years. She has been driven by a strong desire to motivate and inspire women to reach their full potential.

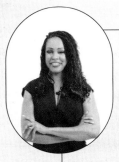

NEIA PRICE-SELMON

Founder and CEO of Wink Studios LLC, Neia Price-Selmon has been a licensed eyelash extension technician and eyelash instructor since 2012. With the eyelash industry continuing to grow and showing no signs of stopping, she opened Wink Studios Lash Academy in 2018, located in Arlington, TX. Neia has a vast knowledge of the industry, with specialties in lash extension health and safety procedures. Working with other eyelash professionals and cosmetology school owners, she has developed an in-depth understanding of which materials and application methods are essential for the education and training of modern eyelash extension application.

Thank You

Milady recognizes, with gratitude and respect, the many professionals who have offered their time to contribute to this edition of *Milady Advanced Services: Eyelashes* and wishes to extend enormous thanks to the cosmetologists, estheticians, schools, and product suppliers who have played an invaluable role in the creation of this edition—not to mention the many reviewers who have weighed in at all stages of production. Without you this edition could not be what it is.

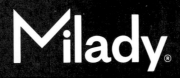

Eyelashes

Advanced Services

Eyelash Extensions

CHAPTER 01

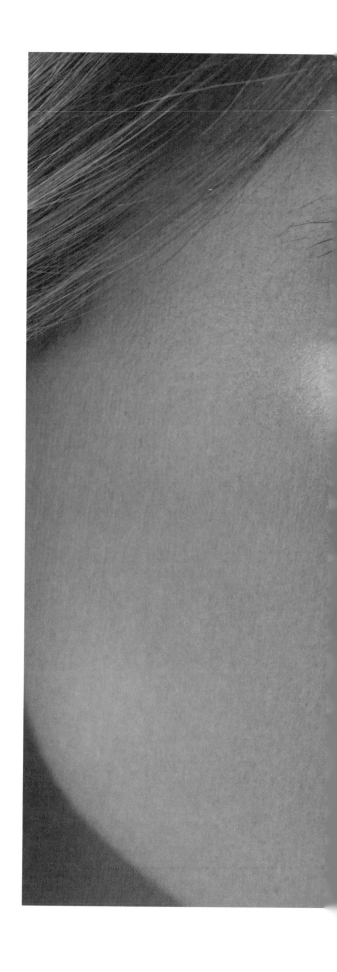

Eyelash Extension History and Careers

🏳 Learning Objectives

After completing this chapter, you will be able to:

1. Explain why it is critical for eyelash technicians to understand the eyelash industry and its history.
2. Identify important historical moments in the use of eyelash enhancements and artificial lashes.
3. Outline the scope of practice for an eyelash technician.
4. Summarize the current and future state of the eyelash industry.

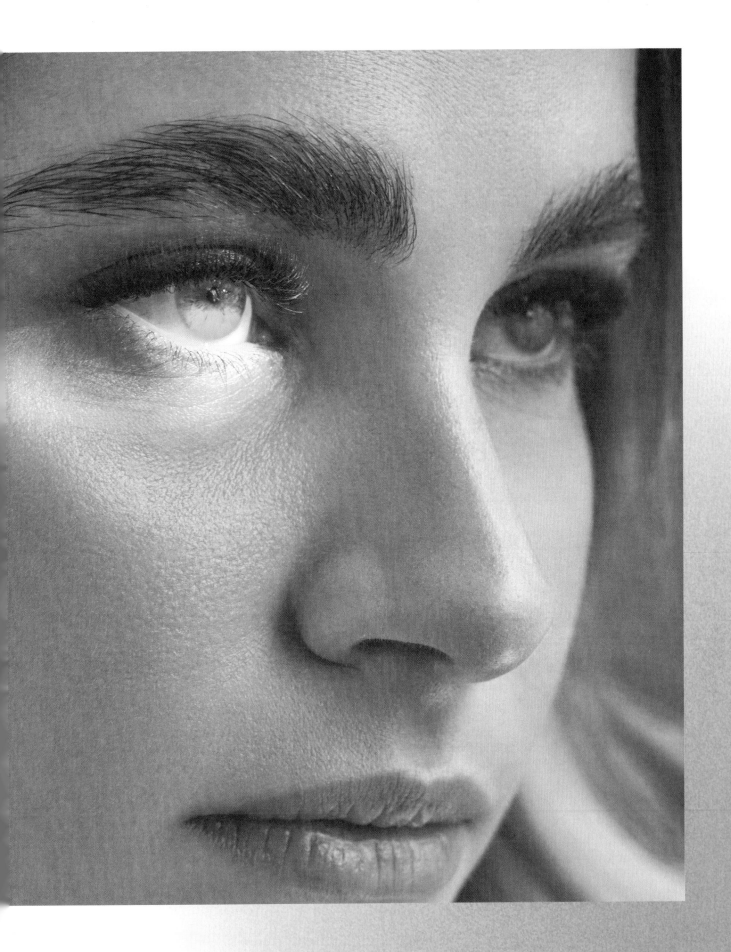

CHAPTER 01
Eyelash Extension History and Careers

Why Study Eyelash Extension History and Careers?

 Learning Objective 01

Explain why it is critical for eyelash technicians to understand the eyelash industry and its history.

Although procedures, products, and styles have changed, eye, eyelash, and eyebrow enhancements have been a part of beautification for thousands of years. Artificial lashes as we know them may have existed for a fraction of this time, but eyelash extensions themselves are over 100 years old, with their own history of innovation and cultural influence. Knowledge of the evolution of eye enhancements will help **eyelash technicians** understand and appreciate the trends of today, including their own place in this growing industry.

Eyelash technicians should study and have a thorough understanding of eyelash extension history and careers because:

- Many older methods of eye, eyelash, and eyebrow enhancement have evolved into techniques still used today.
- Knowing eyelash extension history helps you understand beauty trends and their origins.
- It's important to recognize the limits of the eyelash technician's scope of practice.
- You'll discover the promising career path available to you within the eyelash industry.

 Check In

1. Why is it important to you to study eyelash extension history and careers?

History of Eyelash Enhancements

 Learning Objective 02

Identify important historical moments in the use of eyelash enhancements and artificial lashes.

Many modern beauty practices—including those for eyes and eyelashes—are rooted in our history. The techniques started in ancient cultures developed throughout time to become a part of the beauty industry we know today.

Early Beginnings

Ancient Egyptian men and women would darken their eyelashes using ointments and line their eyes with kohl **(Figure 1-1)**. Ancient Egyptians are credited with creating kohl makeup—originally made from a mixture of ground galena (a black mineral), sulfur, and animal fat—to heavily line the eyes, alleviate eye inflammation, and protect the eyes from the sun's glare. Women also used malachite, a green-colored mineral. Kohl and other ointments were kept in jars complete with application tools **(Figure 1-2)**.

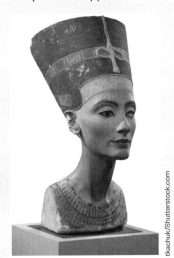

Fig. 1-1: Bust of Nefertiti with kohl-lined eyes.

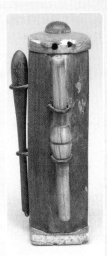

Fig. 1-2: Kohl tube and stick.

Ancient Romans believed that women's lashes should be long and thick. Pliny the Elder, a Roman philosopher, even proclaimed that long, thick lashes were evidence of chastity.[1] Like the Ancient Egyptians, Roman women would use kohl to enhance their eyelashes **(Figure 1-3)**. Other materials used to darken and lengthen eyelashes included burnt cork, soot, and antimony.

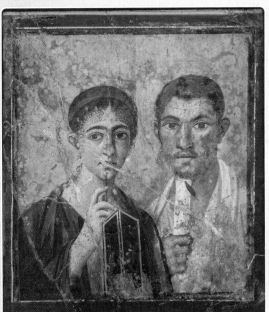

Fig. 1-3: Portrait of a Roman woman with darkened eyes and her husband.

Ch. 01: Eyelash Extension History and Careers

During the Middle Ages, women would take steps to emphasize their forehead. They would remove not only hair from their hairline but also their eyebrows and eyelashes **(Figure 1-4)**.

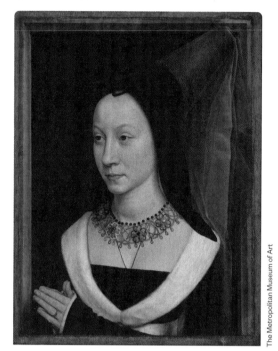

Fig. 1-4: Painting of a woman from the Middle Ages.

The Elizabethan Era brought focus back to the eyebrows and eyelashes. Queen Elizabeth I inspired women to dye their hair red, including their eyebrows and eyelashes **(Figure 1-5)**. Unfortunately, the dyes used were toxic and caused hair loss. Women would alternatively use soot and crushed berries to darken their eyelashes.

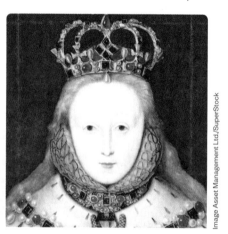

Fig. 1-5: Queen Elizabeth I.

Cosmetics became popular in the Victorian Era. Many women used homemade products, such as soot and tar, to enhance their features. Eugene Rimmel, Queen Victoria's perfumer, developed the first mascara **(Figure 1-6)**. There are also reports of women having hairs sewn onto their eyelids in Paris.

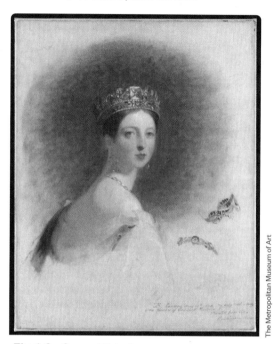

Fig. 1-6: Queen Victoria.

Twentieth-Century Inventions

The early twentieth century saw greater societal acceptance of women's roles outside the home. As women began to frequent department stores and hold jobs, demand for commercial beauty products started to grow. The invention of motion pictures coincided with an abrupt shift in American attitudes. As viewers saw pictures of flawless complexions, beautiful hairstyles, and manicured nails, standards of beauty changed to include these new aspirations. Beauty applications now began to follow trends set by celebrities and society figures.

The twentieth century also saw an explosion of inventions and developments in the expanding beauty industry. Some standouts for eyelash enhancements are summarized in **Table 1-1**.

Table 1-1	Early-Twentieth-Century Eyelash Enhancement Inventions
1902	Karl Nessler patents a method of manufacturing artificial eyebrows and eyelashes in which human hair is attached to isinglass, made from fish skin bladders. These later evolved into Nestolashes and were made of natural hair, artificial hair, or mohair glued to isinglass, silk, or gauze. Although these false eyelashes could be applied at home with supplied adhesive, beauty salons offered application as a service.
1911	Anna Taylor, a Canadian inventor, patents "artificial eyelashes" in the United States.
1916	Director D.W. Griffith films the movie *Intolerance*, in which he requested actor Seena Owen wear dramatic false eyelashes. A wigmaker was hired to weave human hair onto gauze strips, which were then applied to the actor using spirit gum.
1917	T.L. Williams develops and produces what later becomes known as the first modern-day mascara, a mixture of petroleum jelly and coal dust. He later names his makeup brand Maybelline, after his sister.
1931	William Mcdonell invents the first eyelash curler, Kurlash.
1950s	Artificial lashes are made with thin plastic as opposed to human hair and fabric.
1958	Revlon launches the first tube mascara applied with a spiral wand, rather than a cake applied with a brush.

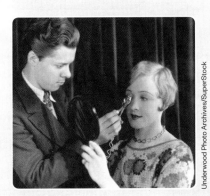

These events paved the way for other leaders in the cosmetics industry. Today, you'll find a wide range of differently formulated mascaras and false eyelash strip styles. Innovations, as well as celebrity and social media influence, continue to drive the ever-changing landscape of eyelash products. For example, although not as common as glue-on strip lashes, magnetic lash strips were patented in 2014 by Katy Stoka, the founder of One Two Cosmetics.

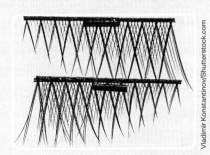

Modern Eyelash Extensions

Beginning in the 1980s, innovators developed semi-permanent eyelash extensions, a more long-term alternative to false strips. Introduced in the United Stated in the early 2000s, this method consisted of applying clusters of lashes onto the client's natural lashes. Methods evolved to where synthetic, single eyelash extensions were affixed to the client's natural lashes. There were, however, several issues with this innovation that impacted sales of the service. These included:

- the use of industrial-grade adhesive and poor-quality extensions,
- lash extension loss, which required clients to return frequently, and
- a long, inconvenient application time.

Modern eyelash extensions are still composed of single hairs attached to the existing eyelashes, but now using a medical-grade adhesive.

Check In

2. What did Ancient Egyptians use to line their eyes, and what was its purpose beyond aesthetics?

3. Who produced the first modern-day mascara?

4. What improvements were made to modern eyelash extensions for durability?

Workbook Assessment

Matching

For the following questions, match each statement to the correct letter choice.

QUESTION 1:

Match the ancient civilizations with the type of eyelash makeup or cosmetic procedures used in those civilizations.

............) ancient Egyptian civilization

............) ancient Roman civilization

............) Middle Ages

............) Elizabethan Era

............) Victorian Era

Choices

A. used burnt cork, soot, and antimony to darken and lengthen eyelashes

B. used soot and crushed berries to darken eyelashes

C. used a mixture of ground galena, sulfur, and animal fat to line the eyes

D. applied soot and tar to enhance features

E. removed hair from eyelashes and eyebrows

QUESTION 2:

Match the eyelash enhancement inventions of the first half of the twentieth century with their inventors.

............) patented a method for manufacturing artificial eyebrows and eyelashes in which human hair is attached to isinglass

............) developed the first modern-day mascara made from a mixture of petroleum jelly and coal dust

............) patented "artificial eyelashes" in the United States

............) invented the first eyelash curler, Kurlash

............) requested actor Seena Owen to wear dramatic false eyelashes in the movie *Intolerance*

Choices

A. William McDonell

B. Karl Nessler

C. D.W. Griffith

D. T.L. Williams

E. Anna Taylor

Scope of Practice and Laws

Learning Objective 03
Outline the scope of practice for an eyelash technician.

Eyelash technician licensing, certification, and governing laws vary widely by state. With this license, eyelash technicians are at base able to receive compensation for applying eyelash extensions—eyelash lifts or perms and color tints depend on your state's regulations. Historically, these services have been performed by estheticians or cosmetologists with proper training and a certification. The objective and priority of eyelash technicians is to safely enhance the appearance of the natural lashes while maintaining their health and integrity.

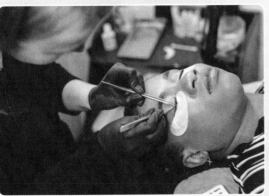
Gustavo Fring/Pexels.com

Caution!
Check with your state board for procedures you're allowed to perform with an eyelash extension certification or licensure. Be sure to confirm what eyelash and eyebrow services are covered under your existing cosmetology or esthetics license, if applicable.

Eyelash technicians must know how to avoid infections and maintain a safe, clean, and comfortable environment for clients. They must also prioritize educating clients on proper home care to prevent developing infections. To do this, technicians must have knowledge of anatomy and physiology of the eye, common infections and diseases of the eye, and what to do in case of emergency. They must know about the lash cycle, how to adapt procedures to client needs, and how to safely remove lashes with approved products. Improper training or incorrect application of infection control practices may result in injury, infections, and the spread of communicable diseases.

The impact of the eyelash technician scope of practice includes:

- With proper training, an eyelash technician will see lashes that may indicate the person should be advised to see a medical professional, such as buildup of makeup or sebum, dust and debris, or evidence of parasitic infestation.
- In most states, eyelash technicians must be either a medical professional or a licensed cosmetologist or esthetician. If a person does not live in a state that issues a specific eyelash technician license, they must choose between completing a training program in cosmetology or esthetics.
- Eyelash technicians following their state's regulations and procedures will give more credibility to the profession, garner higher wages, and provide overall better oversight of infection control and health practices to better protect the public, as well as eyelash technicians themselves.

By knowing the scope of their practice, eyelash technicians will make better choices for their education, services, and performance of their infection control duties, as well as knowing what they can and cannot legally offer their clients. Check your state board for the rules and regulations that affect you.

Check In
5. What is the main objective of an eyelash technician?

Ch. 01: Eyelash Extension History and Careers

Workbook Assessment

Please circle the correct answer for each question below.

Multiple Choice

QUESTION 3:

Which of the following statements is true of eyelash technician licensing laws?

A) They are directly governed by the federal government.

B) They vary widely by state.

C) They require a person to have a medical degree at the minimum to become an eyelash technician.

D) They regulate liability but do not establish minimum requirements to become an eyelash technician.

QUESTION 4:

Samina is certified as an eyelash technician and has worked for three years at a local salon as an eyelash technician. Samina is thinking about moving to another state and looking for a job as an eyelash technician there. Which of the following is true in the given scenario?

A) Samina may not be eligible to work as an eyelash technician in another state with her current certification.

B) Samina can work as an eyelash technician anywhere in the United States, so long as she has a certification from one of the states.

C) Samina may administer eyelash lifts or perms in any state but not eyelash extensions.

D) Samina can administer eyelash color tints in any other state but not eyelash extensions.

QUESTION 5:

What is the primary objective of eyelash technicians?

A) to safely enhance the appearance of the natural lashes while maintaining their health and integrity

B) to identify, diagnose, and treat eye infections prior to administering any cosmetic treatment

C) to administer cosmetic procedures such as dermal filling and eyelifts

D) to teach clients how to enhance the shape of their eyes using makeup techniques

---

QUESTION 6:

Why is an understanding of the scope of practice important for eyelash technicians?

A) It helps technicians establish a client base.

B) It helps technicians obtain waivers from their clients and reduce liability in case of malpractice.

C) It helps technicians become better at their skill.

D) It helps technicians make better choices for their education and services.

QUESTION 7:

Nimai's mother Fatima is a certified eyelash technician. Nimai has spent many years watching Fatima apply eyelash extensions to clients. Nimai also applies their own eyelash extensions using do-it-yourself kits and wants to work as an eyelash extension technician in Fatima's salon. Which of the following is true in the given scenario?

A) Nimai has more training over the years than most people and, therefore, may work in the salon.

B) Nimai must complete a training program and acquire the required license or certificate before working in the salon.

C) Nimai must gain experience by applying eyelash extensions to others and then start working in the salon.

D) Nimai may work in the salon and receive on-the-job training under Fatima before they can start applying eyelash extensions on their own.

QUESTION 8:

With proper training, which of the following will eyelash technicians be able to do?

A) They will be able to spot a buildup of sebum and advise the client to see a medical professional.

B) They will be able to spot and treat parasitic infestation in the eyelashes.

C) They will be able to offer advice to clients on the type of eyeglasses or contact lenses they need.

D) They will be able to administer basic vision therapy such as eye exercises.

QUESTION 9:

If a person lives in a state that does not issue a specific eyelash technician license, which of the following must they do to be able to practice as an eyelash technician?

A) They must choose another specialty or move to another state to complete an eyelash technician licensing program.

B) They must apprentice under another certified technician from another state.

C) They must complete a licensing program in cosmetology or esthetics, depending on state board licensure requirements.

D) They must complete a premed course.

QUESTION 10:

Which of the following actions by eyelash technicians is most likely to increase the credibility of the profession?

A) establishing upscale salons

B) offering eyelash services that clients want even if technicians are not certified to offer them

C) following the state's regulations and procedures

D) offering more expensive alternative products and procedures than required

---

QUESTION 11:

Which of the following is most likely to be an outcome of eyelash technicians following their state's regulations and procedures?

A) superior skill development of the technicians

B) lower wages because of the inability to provide a wide range of services

C) increased liability of the salon

D) provision of overall better oversight of infection control practices

Overview of the Eyelash Industry

 Learning Objective 04

Summarize the current and future state of the eyelash industry.

If you have dreams to become an eyelash artist with your own studio, understanding the future of the industry will help you be realistic about your place in it. The industry is expected to reach $1.5 billion in annual product sales by 2023.[2] Consumers rely on professionals to achieve their own personalized eyelash extension look, provide them with products to care for their eyelash extensions, and guarantee a specific outcome after an appointment.[3]

 Did You Know?

Career options are not limited to being a lash artist! With certification or licensure, you could also be a shop or studio owner, eyelash extension educator, or a product salesperson.

Receiving eyelash services becomes a regular routine like haircoloring or facials. While women make up most of the client base, men do represent a small portion. Fifty percent of all clients fall within the 18 to 34 age range.

The eyelash enhancement industry shows no signs of slowing down over the next 5- to 10-year period. Sixty-three percent of those employed in the eyelash extension industry say that they are earning what they expected when they took their job.[4] As trends continue to point to the resiliency of personal services, the health-and-beauty segment is itself primed for significant growth in years to come. According to a recent report, the global personal care services market is expected to reach $488.9 billion by 2025.[5] All told, the field looks very promising for any students, cosmetologists, or estheticians wanting to build a niche for themselves.

Eyelash technicians are in high demand. There are lash salon owners across the world charging up to $400 per lash service, or leasing spaces to technicians to do the same. The average technician who performs a minimum of five procedures per week and charges $150 per procedure could earn as much as $39,000 per year, with that number increasing with higher fees per service or more procedures per week. Considering that the average client who has received a professional eyelash extension application will visit their preferred venue once every 4 to 6 weeks to maintain their eyelash extension services, the prospects for the enterprising eyelash technician are looking very nice indeed.[6]

 Check In

6. What is the most common demographic for eyelash extensions?

7. How often does the average eyelash extension client come in for a service?

Workbook Assessment

Multiple Choice

Please circle the correct answer for each question below.

QUESTION 12:

The eyelash industry is expected to reach _____ in annual product sales by 2023.

    A) $10 million

    B) $500 million

    C) $1.5 billion

    D) $488.9 billion

QUESTION 13:

Which of the following is true of the eyelash industry?

    A) Getting eyelashes done is becoming a routine like hair coloring or facials.

    B) Getting lashes done is largely limited to celebrities and public figures.

    C) Contrary to the common conception, men make up most of the clientele.

    D) People rarely revisit a salon once they have had their eyelash extensions done.

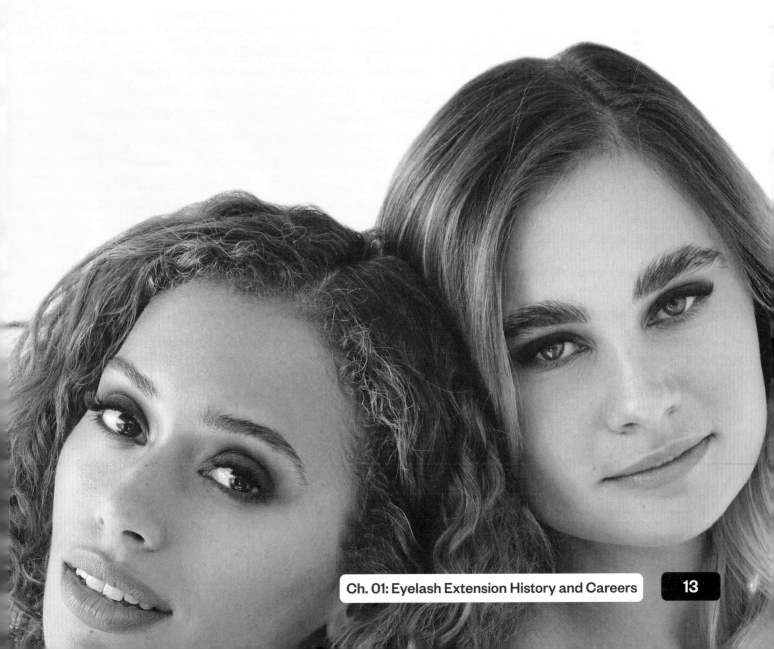

Ch. 01: Eyelash Extension History and Careers

QUESTION 14:

Which of the following demographics makes up half of the clientele in the eyelash industry?

A) people within the 18 to 34 age range

B) adolescents within the 15 to 18 age range

C) working women within the 35 to 45 age range

D) people within the 45 to 60 age range

QUESTION 15:

In the context of the future of eyelash services, which of the following statements is true of the eyelash services market?

A) Most eyelash technicians do not earn what they expected to earn when they started their job.

B) The prospects for lash technicians are very good as the eyelash enhancement industry is growing.

C) With the advent of do-it-yourself kits, technicians are in less demand than they were a few years ago.

D) The global personal care services market has reached its peak and become stagnant.

QUESTION 16:

Chen wants to become an eyelash technician and wants to join a training program to obtain a license. Chen is uncertain about the future of the eyelash enhancement industry and wants to know more about the prospects in the industry. Chen speaks to their neighbor Tahin, who has been the owner of a successful salon for 15 years. What is Tahin most likely to say to Chen?

A) Chen should pursue the program as it is a fast-growing market.

B) Chen should try out the program but know that most technicians end up earning much less than they expected.

C) Chen should not expect much increase in earnings as that is unlikely to happen.

D) Chen should opt for the program if Chen's plan is to work for salons rather than becoming a business owner.

QUESTION 17:

Cruz, who had gotten eyelash extensions two years ago, takes good care of the extensions and regularly visits an eyelash salon for the maintenance of the extensions. How often do you think Cruz visits the salon for lash service?

A) once every six to eight months

B) once every year

C) once every four to six weeks

D) once every week

Chapter Glossary

eyelash technicians	p. 004	beauty professionals who perform eyelash extension services to enhance the appearance of the natural lashes while maintaining the health and integrity of the lashes
AI-lash tek-**NI**-shun		

Eye and Eyelash Anatomy and Physiology

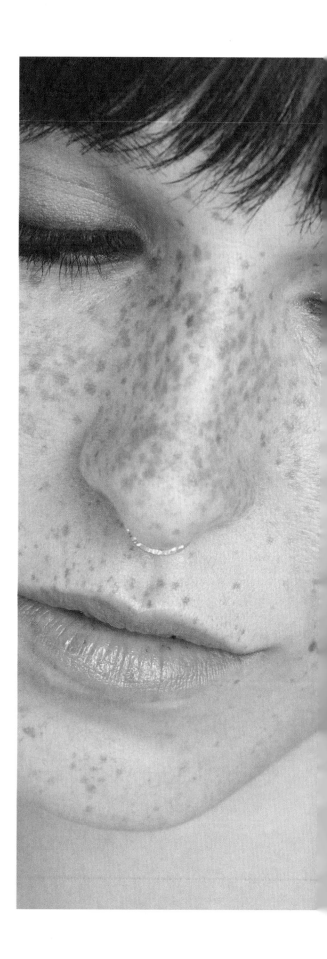

🏳 Learning Objectives

After completing this chapter, you will be able to:

1. Explain why eyelash technicians need knowledge of eye and eyelash anatomy and physiology.
2. Describe the structures of the eye and their functions.
3. Identify different eye and eyelid shapes.
4. Identify different spacings of the eye on the face.
5. Recognize the growth stages of eyelash hair.

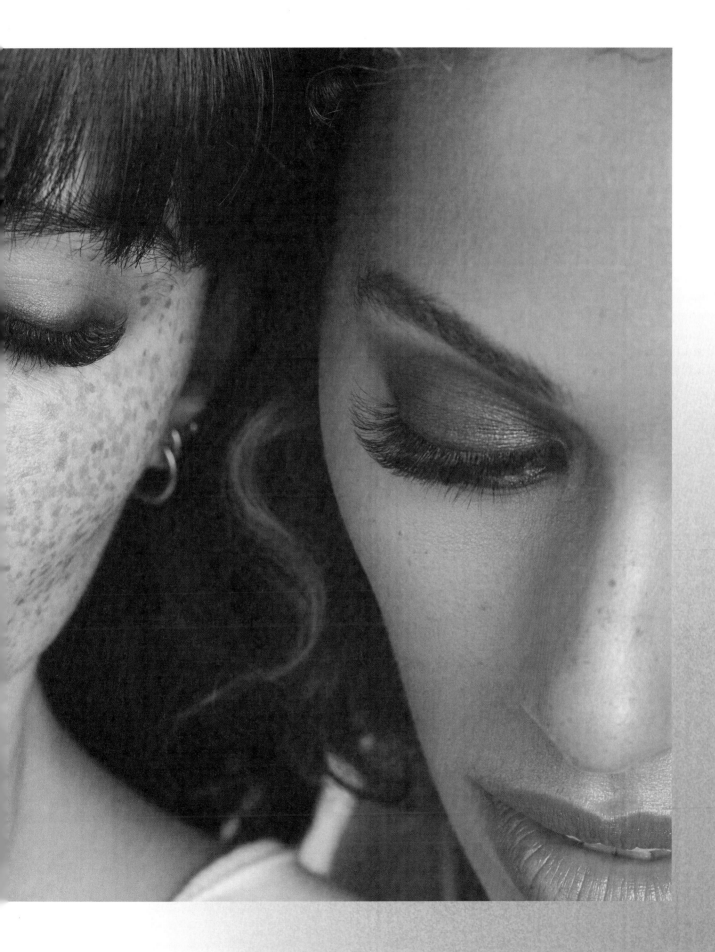

CHAPTER 02

Eye and Eyelash Anatomy and Physiology

Why Study Anatomy and Physiology of the Eye?

 Learning Objective 01

Explain why eyelash technicians need knowledge of eye and eyelash anatomy and physiology.

Eyelash and eyebrow services affect the orbital region of the head, a complex area home to two very sensitive organs of the body and central to human expression and communication. Knowledge of the structure and function of the eyes, eyelids, eyelashes, and eyebrows is critical to be able to protect the health of the eye while still performing beautiful, proportioned services.

Eyelash technicians should have a thorough understanding of eye and eyelash anatomy and physiology because:

- The more technicians understand about eye structure and function, the safer, better experiences they can provide for their clients.
- Failing to work with the client's anatomy can have disastrous results, ranging from discomfort to blindness in the worst case.
- Eyelash services must be modified to fit the client's eye shape and spacing. Lashes are not a one-size-fits-all service!
- Successful eyelash services take into account the hair growth cycle of eyelashes, protecting the growing lash and giving the best final look.

 Check In

1. Why do you think it is important to understand eye and eyelash anatomy and physiology?

Anatomy of the Eye

 Learning Objective 02

Describe the structures of the eye and their functions.

The eye is a complex, sensitive organ made up of several protective structures **(Figure 2–1)**. Although our focus is on the lash, we must still understand the healthy function of the entire orbital region. This includes the eyelids and eyebrows, which along with the eyelashes exist to protect the eye from harmful substances or objects.

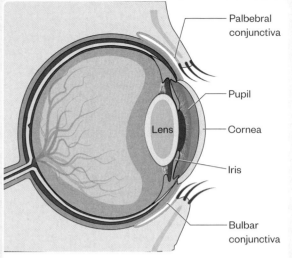

Fig. 2-1: Anatomy of the eye.

The Eye

Starting at the outermost layer, the eye is protected by the **conjunctiva**, a thin, clear, moist mucous membrane that coats the inner surface of the eyelids and outer surface of the eye. The part of the conjunctiva covering the eye's white surface, or the *sclera*, is known as the *bulbar conjunctiva* (or *ocular conjunctiva*). The *palpebral conjunctiva* covers the inside of the eyelid and can be seen when the lid is pulled slightly away from the eye. Both membranes lubricate and protect the eye, preventing microbes from entering.

Next, the transparent **cornea** covers and protects the iris, pupil, lens, anterior chamber, and other internal structures. In addition to offering physical and microbial protection, the cornea also reflects light and assists considerably in focusing the eye. Think of the cornea like a camera lens, sending clear images back to the retina. The cornea is very sensitive to touch, has many layers, and is packed with 70 to 80 sensory nerves. Because the cornea lacks its own blood supply, the *aqueous humor* (fluid) inside the eye provides nutrients and stabilizes the eye's pressure, while tears produced by the *lacrimal gland* lubricate and clean its outside. Healthy tear films are vital to the cornea, keeping the eye moist, protecting it from infections, and healing wounds.

The Eyelids

The **eyelids** are thin coverings of skin that protect the eye. They spread tears through continuous blinking, keeping the cornea and conjunctiva moist. This barrier keeps our eyes from drying out while we sleep, as well as clearing debris and dust when we blink. The edge of the eyelid is home to two types of glands: **glands of Zeis** at the end of the eyelash follicle and **meibomian glands** at the back of the eyelid **(Figure 2–2)**. There are about 50 glands on the upper and 25 on the lower eyelid. These sebaceous glands produce oil that helps prevent evaporation of the tear film and keep tears from spilling onto the cheeks.

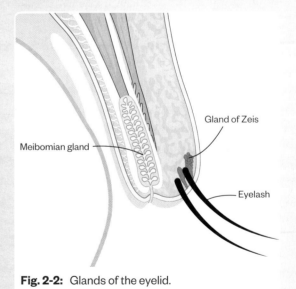

Fig. 2-2: Glands of the eyelid.

The Eyelashes

Eyelashes are the hairs that grow at the edge of the eyelids. A human eye has 75 to 80 lashes on the lower eyelid and 90 to 160 on the upper eyelid, with some eyelids having several rows of lashes.[1] The eyelashes act like a broom, sweeping away debris before it enters the eye. Eyelashes sense when a foreign object gets too close, causing a blink reflex that both bats away danger and creates a physical barrier to the eye. When the eye is open, eyelashes act as a passive filter, making it harder for airborne particles to fall into the surface of the eye.

The Eyebrows

Eyebrows are arched lines of hair that grow on the skin along the brow bone above the eye socket. The eyebrows protect the eyes from sun and dust, as well as direct moisture away from the eyes. Brows also play an important role in expressing emotions and being able to recognize human faces.[2] An eyebrow can be broken down into three areas, moving from the center of the face outward: head, body, and tail **(Figure 2-3)**. The hair in each section usually grows in a different direction—upward (head), diagonally or sideways (body), and downward (tail)—to help the eyebrow fulfill its protective functions. Working with this differing hair growth will be important during brow chemical services.

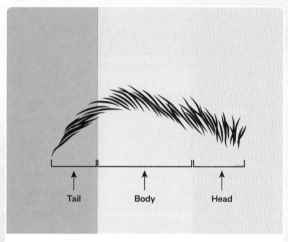

Fig. 2-3: Sections of the eyebrow.

Check In

2. What does the conjunctiva do?

3. How do the eyelashes protect the eye?

Workbook Assessment

Please circle the correct answer for each question below.

Multiple Choice

QUESTION 1:
The thin, clear, moist mucous membrane that coats the inner surface of the eyelids and the outer surface of the eye is called the ....

A) conjunctiva

B) cornea

C) sclera

D) iris

QUESTION 2:
Zindel experiences eye irritation and blurry vision. After examining Zindel's eyes, the doctor explains to Zindel that the covering that protects the internal structures of the eye has become inflamed. This covering also acts like a camera lens and sends clear images back to the retina. Which part of the eye is the doctor referring to in the given scenario?

A) the *aqueous humor*

B) the *palpebral conjunctiva*

C) the *sclera*

D) the *cornea*

QUESTION 3:
Which of the following is a function of the cornea?

A) It secretes tears to lubricate the eye.

B) It provides nutrition to the eye.

C) It assists in focusing the eye.

D) It stabilizes the eye's pressure.

QUESTION 4:
What are the thin coverings of skin that protect the eye called?

A) sebaceous glands

B) lacrimal glands

C) the eyelids

D) the eyelashes

QUESTION 5:
What is the role of tear films in the eyes?

A) to keep the eyes moist and heal wounds

B) to keep tears from spilling onto the cheeks

C) to prevent the evaporation of the oil secreted by sebaceous glands

D) to reflect light and assist in focusing the eye

QUESTION 6:
Identify a difference between glands of Zeis and meibomian glands.

A) Glands of Zeis are sebaceous glands, whereas meibomian glands are tear glands.

B) Glands of Zeis secrete tears, whereas meibomian glands secrete oil.

C) Glands of Zeis are located at the end of the eyelash follicles, whereas meibomian glands are located at the back of the eyelids.

D) Glands of Zeis are located at the lateral ends of the eye orbit, whereas meibomian glands are located at the end of the eyelash follicles.

QUESTION 7:

Which of the following statements is true of the distribution of sebaceous glands in the eye?

A) They are present on the upper eyelid but not on the lower eyelid.

B) There are about 50 sebaceous glands on the upper eyelid.

C) There are approximately 500 sebaceous glands in each eyelid.

D) Sebaceous glands are confined to the back of the eyelids.

QUESTION 8:

Nuria opens a box full of old books. The moment the box opens, it releases a plume of dust. Which of the following parts of Nuria's eyes will quickly sense the dust in the air and cause a blink reflex to create a barrier between the eyes and dust?

A) the eyelashes

B) the iris

C) the *aqueous humor*

D) the *palpebral conjunctiva*

QUESTION 9:

Which of the following statements is true of the eyebrows?

A) They prevent microbes from entering the eyes.

B) They control the amount of light that enters the pupil.

C) They are exclusively aesthetic and not functional.

D) They play an important role in expressing emotions.

QUESTION 10:

When you exercise or when the weather is hot and your body perspires to cool you off, which of the following prevents the sweat from your forehead from falling into your eyes?

A) the eyebrows

B) the conjunctiva

C) glands of Zeis

D) meibomian glands

Eye and Eyelid Shapes

 Learning Objective 03

Identify different eye and eyelid shapes.

People naturally have a variety of eye and eyelid shapes. An important part of your consultation process will be identifying what features you are working with **(Table 2–1)**—working with the shape of your client's eyes can make or break your set depending on your client's desired finished look. You can then create a plan that uses eyelash extensions and/or eye makeup to alter the shape and spacing of the eyes. Your work can open, elongate, and bring balance to the face, accenting your client's features.

Table 2-1 Eye and Eyelid Shapes

Shapes				Description
				Almond Eyes have equal proportions with visible lid. Opt for a pair of wispy, voluminous lashes. For added flair, go for lashes that are tapered or longer on the outer corners.
				Round Eye width and height are equal; eyes appear large and bright. To accentuate the eye, go for long, tapered lashes that are longer at the ends, such as cat eyelashes (short to long lash line). Avoid short curly lashes to keep the eye from looking rounder.
				Downturned Eyes have a slight drop on the outer corners, turning downward and sitting lower than the inner corner. Use D or DD curl on the outer corner lashes to give the illusion that the eye is lifted.
				Upturned Outer corners of the eyes turn upward and are higher than the inner corner. To balance the eye out and give the illusion that the eye is sitting straight, go flatter on the ends with B or C curls.
				Monolid Eyelids have no crease. Use medium-length lashes no longer than 12 mm, usually with L or L+ curl, to give the illusion of a creased lid.
				Hooded Eyes have a droopy over crease, making the lid look smaller. Longer curly lashes work best to minimize the veil of skin that droops over the crease, while bringing the focus upward toward the brow bone.

*See Chapter 5 Tools, Products, and Ingredients for information on eyelash extension curls, diameter, and length.

 Here's a Tip

To minimize a lazy eye, use a lash that is a bit more curled than the other eye to give the illusion that both eyes are even. For example, using a C curl on one eye and a D curl on the other will help balance the eyes and soften the difference between them.

Ch. 02: Eye and Eyelash Anatomy and Physiology

Check In

4. Name the six different eye and eyelid shapes.

Workbook Assessment

Matching

For the following questions, match each statement to the correct letter choice.

QUESTION 11:

Match the names of the eye types with their descriptions.

………….) Eyes have equal proportions with visible lid.

………….) Eyes have a droopy over crease, making the lid look smaller.

………….) Eye width and height are equal.

………….) Outer corners of the eyes are higher than the inner corners.

………….) Eyes have a slight drop on the outer corners.

………….) Eyelids have no crease.

Choices

A. upturned eyes
B. round eyes
C. downturned eyes
D. monolid eyes
E. almond-shaped eyes
F. hooded eyes

QUESTION 12:

Match the recommended type of lashes to the corresponding eye types.

............) hooded eyes

............) almond-shaped eyes

............) downturned eyes

............) round eyes

............) monolid eyes

............) upturned eyes

Choices

A. wispy, voluminous lashes

B. long, tapered lashes that are longer at the ends

C. long curly lashes

D. medium-length lashes no longer than 12 mm, usually with L or L+ curl

E. use B or C curls at the ends

F. D or DD curl on the outer corner lashes

Eye Spacing on the Face

Learning Objective 04

Identify different spacings of the eye on the face.

As with eye and eyelid shape, a key part of the consultation is determining the spacing of your client's eyes on their face **(Table 2-2)**. Are the eyes wide apart? Close together? Prominent or deep set? This information will help determine the type of lash you should use to offset the spacing and flatter your client.

Table 2-2 — Eye Spacing

				Prominent (protruding) Eyes have the appearance of bulging out of the eye socket. Use short to medium lashes that are not super curly. A mixture of B and C curls will avoid overpowering the eyes and making them look more protruding.
				Deep set Eyes set deep into skull with more prominent brow bone. Go for a wispy mixture of short and long lashes with extra length and even a CC or D curl. This will draw the focus from the brow bone to the center of the eyes.
				Close set Space between the eyes is *less than* the width of one eye. Go longer on the ends, usually with a cat-eye style, to give the illusion that the eyes are further apart.
				Wide set Space between the eyes is *greater than* the width of one eye. Offset the extra space by using longer lashes until about the center of the lash, then use a similar length all the way through the ends. This will avoid bringing extra attention outward as well.

Ch. 02: Eye and Eyelash Anatomy and Physiology

Facial Shapes

Facial shape is another factor that should be considered when creating the ideal lash map **(Table 2–3)**.

Table 2-3	Face Shapes			
	Oval	Forehead slightly wider than chin	Base lash style on eye shape and eye spacing, as oval face shapes are already balanced.
	Round	Wide at center, round hairline, round chin	Use longer lashes in the center of the eye to lengthen and diminish roundness.
	Square	Wide temples, narrow middle-third of face, squared-off jaw	Use longer lashes in the center of the eye to lengthen and diminish the hard jawline.
	Triangle	Narrow forehead, wide jaw and chin line	Create more width at the forehead by applying long, thick lashes evenly across the eye.
	Oblong	Long, narrow face with hollow cheeks	Create more width by applying longer extensions on the outside corners of the eye.
	Diamond	Narrow forehead, width at cheekbones, narrow chin	Accentuate both diamond and heart-shaped faces by using longer lashes on the outside corner of the eyes or by using long, thick lashes evenly across the eye.
	Heart	Wide forehead, narrow chin line	

Focus On

Competing Focuses

Sometimes you will find that the best eyelash applications for your client's eye shape, spacing, and face shape conflict with one another. In this case, create the lash map that flatters your client's most prominent features. The goal should be to make the client look their best.

For example, for a client with round eyes and a square face, you could either do a cat-eye style or keep the length in the center of the eye. Go for a cat-eye style if the client's round eyes are more noticeable. Conversely, go for length in the center of the eye if the client's square face is more prominent.

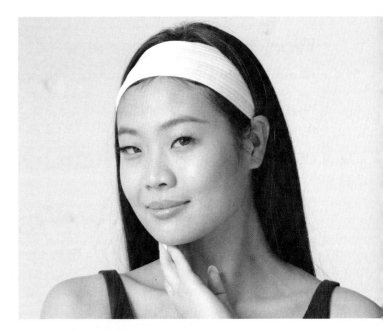

 Check In

5. How should you apply lash extensions to flatter deep-set eyes?

6. How should you apply lash extensions to flatter a square face?

Workbook Assessment

Fill in the blanks below using words from the provided word bank.

Fill in the Blank

QUESTION 13:

.... or protruding eyes have the appearance of bulging out of the eye socket. A short to medium mixture of .... and .... curls is the recommended lash extension for this type of eyes.

QUESTION 14:

Nimsi is evaluating a new client's eye spacing to decide the most suitable style of lash extensions. The client's eyes are set way back into the skull with a prominent looking brow. Nimsi concludes that the client has .... eyes. In this case, Nimsi must go for a wispy mixture of short and long lashes with extra length and a CC or D curl—a style that will draw the focus from the

.... to the ....

QUESTION 15:

The space between .... eyes is less than the width of one eye.

The recommended lash style for this type of eyes is the .... style.

QUESTION 16:

Sabin is planning to get lash extensions. Based on eye spacing, the lash technician tells Sabin that the best style for Sabin's eyes is to use longer lashes until about the center of the lash and then use a similar length all the way through the ends. This will offset the space in the middle without drawing attention outward.

Based on the given information, Sabin most likely has .... eyes.

QUESTION 17:

While evaluating a client's face and eyes to create a lash map, the lash technician concludes that there is no need to consider the face shape in the evaluation as it is already balanced. The client most likely has a(n) .... face shape.

Word Bank

forehead
brow bone
wide-set
center
oval
prominent
wide-set
square
B
triangle
deep-set
cat eye
C
eye
outside
heart
close-set
round

Ch. 02: Eye and Eyelash Anatomy and Physiology

QUESTION 18:

To diminish the circular shape of a .... face shape and lengthen it, a lash technician is likely to apply longer lashes in the .... of the eye.

QUESTION 19:

Dierdre's client has a wide temple with narrow middle-third of face and a pronounced and angular jawline. Based on the face shape, Dierdre applies longer lash extensions in the center of the eye to lengthen and diminish the hard jawline. In the given scenario, the client most likely has a(n) .... face shape.

QUESTION 20:

Yuvi has a narrow forehead and a relatively wider jaw and chin line. In the context of face shapes, Yuvi has a(n) .... face. The lash technician must create more width at the .... by applying long, thick lashes evenly across the eye.

QUESTION 21:

Astrid evaluates a client with an oblong face and prominent eyes. To create more width on the face, Astrid must apply longer extensions on the .... corners of the eye.

QUESTION 22:

Menna has a wide forehead and a narrow chin line. The space between Menna's eyes is greater than the width of one eye. Menna has a(n) .... face shape and .... eyes.

Eyelash Hair Growth Stages

 Learning Objective 05

Recognize the growth stages of eyelash hair.

As with other human hair, the eyelashes follow a growth cycle. Knowing the stages of this cycle is important because this will allow you to select the correct lashes for extension application, ensuring that the extensions look their best and last as long as possible **(Figure 2–4)**.

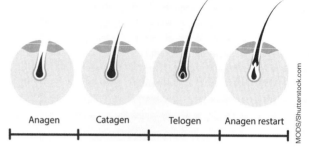

Fig. 2-4: Hair growth-cycle of eyelashes.

Anagen Stage

The **anagen** stage is when lashes are undergoing new growth. This can last about 4 to 7 weeks (30 to 45 days). Application of extensions at this stage is not recommended because they tend to weigh down the natural lashes, which can result in premature detachment. Additionally, lashes applied during the anagen stage will look unnatural once the natural lashes reach full growth. Extensions 8 to 9 mm in length are recommended at this phase.

 Caution!

During the anagen stage, eyelashes are weak, and artificial lashes may put too much weight on them. This can cause damage or slow down lash growth.

Catagen Stage

The **catagen** stage is the transitional stage of hair growth (between anagen and telogen stages) and lasts about 2 to 3 weeks (12 to 21 days). At this stage, the lash has just finished growing. This is the ideal growth stage for extension placement. Artificial lashes applied at this stage will last longer and look more natural than extensions applied during other growth stages. Extensions 10 to 12 mm in length are recommended.

Telogen Stage

The **telogen** stage is the resting stage and can last for up to 14 weeks (100 days). Lash hairs in this stage are at their longest, darkest, and coarsest. This is an acceptable stage for lash placement, although lashes at this stage will be shed more quickly than those applied to lashes in the catagen stage. Extensions 12 to 14 mm in length are recommended.

 Check In

7. During which stage of hair growth are hairs actively growing?

8. What is the best stage of lash growth during which to apply lash extensions?

Workbook Assessment

Please circle the correct answer for each question below.

Multiple Choice

QUESTION 23:

Identify the best stage for the application of eyelash extension in the given illustration of the stages of the eyelash growth cycle.

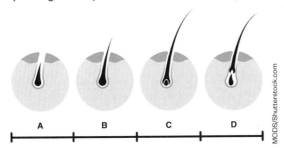

A) A

B) B

C) C

D) D

QUESTION 24:

During the .... stage of the eyelash growth cycle, eyelashes undergo new growth.

A) anagen

B) catagen

C) telogen

D) exogen

QUESTION 25:

Which of the following stages of the eyelash growth cycle starts when the eyelashes have just finished growing?

A) the exogen stage

B) the telogen stage

C) the catagen stage

D) the anagen stage

QUESTION 26:

It is not a good idea to apply eyelash extensions during the anagen stage of the eyelash growth cycle because ....

A) the lashes have just finished growing and are still too weak

B) this stage requires longer than normal eyelash extensions, which does not create a suitable look

C) eyelash extensions applied at this stage get stuck to the natural lashes, making them difficult to remove later

D) eyelash extensions are too heavy for the growing eyelashes

QUESTION 27:

Lin, a lash technician, advises a client, Sabaa, to wait for a few weeks before the application of lash extensions. However, Sabaa wants to get the extensions before leaving for a vacation. Lin applies the lashes. Two weeks later, Sabaa comes back to complain that the extensions are falling out, and the ones that have not fallen out look unnatural. Based on the given information, at what stage of the eyelash growth cycle did Sabaa most likely get the eyelash extensions done?

A) the exogen stage

B) the telogen stage

C) the catagen stage

D) the anagen stage

QUESTION 28:

How long does the catagen stage of the eyelash growth cycle last?

A) 2 to 3 weeks

B) 4 to 7 weeks

C) up to 14 weeks

D) about 24 weeks

QUESTION 29:

Ezra booked an appointment with an eyelash technician for a consultation. After checking the eyelash growth stage, the technician asked Ezra to wait for about 2 weeks before getting extensions as the eyelashes will then enter the growth stage that is best for eyelash extension application. Based on the given information, at the time of consultation, Ezra's eyelashes were in the .... growth stage.

A) exogen

B) telogen

C) catagen

D) anagen

QUESTION 30:

What length of eyelash extensions is recommended for application during the catagen stage of the eyelash growth cycle?

A) 12 to 14 mm

B) 10 to 12 mm

C) 8 to 9 mm

D) 5 to 6 mm

QUESTION 31:

During the .... stage of the eyelash growth cycle, eyelash hairs are at their longest, darkest, and coarsest.

A) anagen

B) catagen

C) anagen restart

D) telogen

QUESTION 32:

Fauzia wants to get eyelash extensions. After examining Fauzia's lashes, the technician tells Fauzia that while extensions can be applied at this stage without damaging the natural eyelashes, this is not the best stage for extension application. The extensions will shed more quickly than usual. Fauzia's eyelashes are most likely in the .... stage of the eyelash growth cycle.

A) telogen

B) anagen

C) catagen

D) exogen

Chapter Glossary

anagen *AN-uh-jen*	p. 030	first stage of hair growth during which new hair is produced and actively growing
catagen *KAT-uh-jen*	p. 030	transitional stage of hair growth between active growth (anagen) and the resting stage (telogen)
conjunctiva *kon-juhngk-TAI-vuh*	p. 019	thin, clear, moist mucous membrane that coats the inner surface of the eyelids and outer surface of the eye
cornea *kor-nee-uh*	p. 019	transparent covering that protects the iris, pupil, lens, anterior chamber, and other internal structures of the eye; plays an important focusing role
eyelashes *AI-la-shuhz*	p. 020	hairs at the edge of the eyelids
eyelids *AI-lidz*	p. 019	thin coverings of skin that protect the eye
glands of Zeis *glandz of zees*	p. 019	sebaceous glands at the end of the eyelash follicle
meibomian glands *may-BOH-me-uhn glandz*	p. 019	sebaceous glands at the back of the eyelid
telogen *TEE-loh-jen*	p. 030	resting stage of hair growth; final phase in the hair cycle that lasts until the fully grown hair is shed

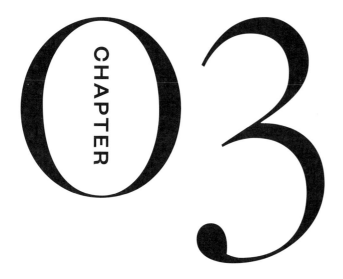

Disorders, Diseases, and Allergies of the Eye Area

🏳 Learning Objectives

After completing this chapter, you will be able to:

1. Explain why eyelash technicians need to understand disorders, diseases, and allergies of the eye area.
2. Recognize disorders and diseases of the eye, eyelid, eyelash, and eyebrow.
3. Identify allergies and sensitivities related to eyelash extensions.

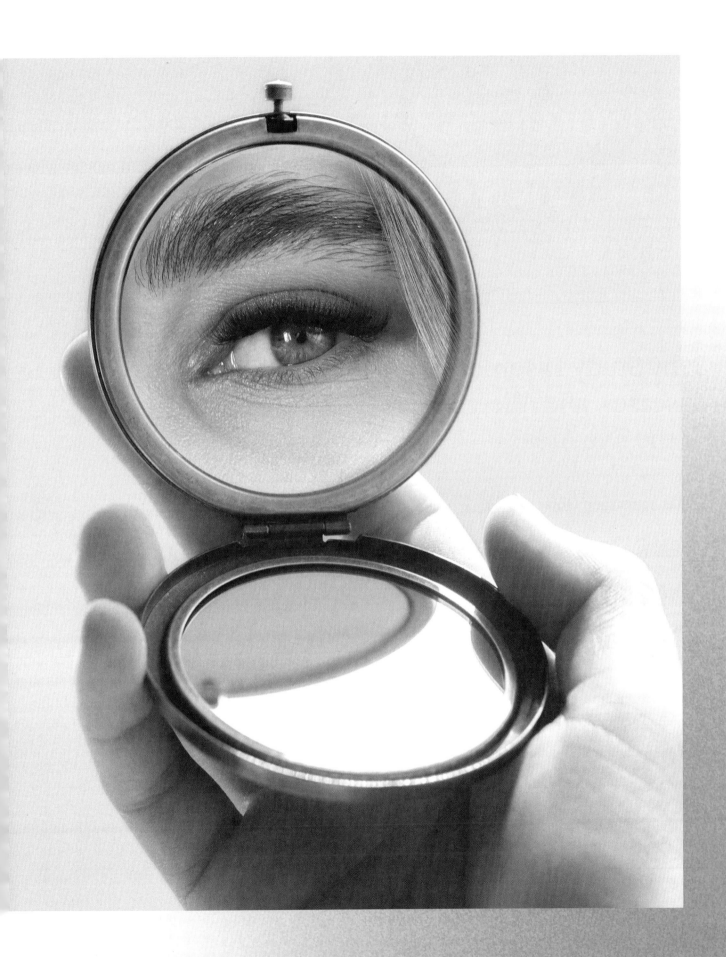

CHAPTER 03

Disorders, Diseases, and Allergies of the Eye Area

Why Study Disorders, Diseases, and Allergies of the Eye Area?

 Learning Objective 01

Explain why eyelash technicians need to understand disorders, diseases, and allergies of the eye area.

Responsible eyelash technicians must understand and be able to recognize the types of eye, eyelid, eyelash, and eyebrow disorders and diseases they may encounter. These disorders are very often contraindications for eyelash and/or eyebrow services, and to work on many of them is to risk spreading a contagious disease to yourself and others. Allergies are another contraindication that you will need to screen and test for before providing services. Although sensitivities can be a contraindication as well, it is important to consider the role that sensitization can have on the longevity of your career as an eyelash technician.

Eyelash technicians should study and have a thorough understanding of disorders, diseases, and allergies of the eye area because:

- Providing eyelash extension services requires an understanding of the eye's structure and common eye-related problems, including potentially contagious disorders and diseases.
- Allergies and sensitivities are common contraindications for eyelash and eyebrow services that should be screened for and patch-tested against prior to performing a service.
- Being able to identify an unexpected adverse reaction early in a service is an important step in responding swiftly and appropriately.

 Check In

1. Why do you think it is important to study disorders, diseases, and allergies of the eye area?

Disorders and Diseases of the Eye Area

 Learning Objective 02

Recognize disorders and diseases of the eye, eyelid, eyelash, and eyebrow.

You should avoid serving a client with an inflamed eye, eyelid, or eyebrow disorder regardless of whether the condition is contagious. Kindly suggest that proper measures be taken to prevent more serious consequences and refer the client to a medical professional.

 Caution!

Remember, eyelash technicians are not allowed to diagnose, treat, or recommend treatments for infections, diseases, or conditions. Refer clients to their healthcare providers.

Blepharitis

Blepharitis, inflammation of the eyelids, is chronically difficult to treat and causes dry eyes with occasional crusting or flakey material on the eyelashes after sleeping **(Figure 3–1)**. Light sensitivity, discomfort, burning eyes, and the sensation of feeling a sharp object in the eye are additional complaints. Blepharitis is commonly caused by staphylococcus but can occur from other causes. It is not contagious and if left untreated, can cause lash loss and may lead to blindness.

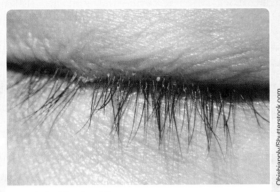

Fig. 3-1: Blepharitis.

Conjunctivitis

Conjunctivitis, also known as *pinkeye*, is an eye infection and may be caused by a bacterium or a virus. It is characterized by burning, red swollen lids, excessive tears, irritation, discomfort, crusted eyelids, discharge from the tear duct, and a gritty feeling in the eyes **(Figure 3–2)**. Bacterial or viral conjunctivitis are very contagious. The bacterial form can be treated with antibiotics; however, the viral form must run its course.

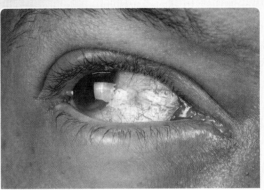

Fig. 3-2: Allergic conjunctivitis.

ALLERGIC CONJUNCTIVITIS

Allergic conjunctivitis is an inflammation of the conjunctiva due to chemical irritants such as shampoos, dirt, smoke, pool chlorine, pollen, perfume, and cosmetics. Allergic conjunctivitis is not contagious, and it usually subsides with the help of eye drops.

Ch. 03: Disorders, Diseases, and Allergies of the Eye Area

Demodex

Demodex refers to a group of microscopic mites that burrow into and live inside the eyelash hair follicle (**Figure 3–3**). These mites will cause the eyelash hair to become loose if too many mites burrow into the same follicle, causing eyelash loss and potentially blindness. Demodex infestation can be the result of dirty, unkept lashes or untreated blepharitis, and it occurs more often in older adults and those with compromised immune systems. Demodex is contagious.

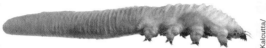

Fig. 3-3: Demodex.

Stye

A **stye** is an inflammation of a Zeis or meibomian gland that appears as a painful, red bump on the eyelid (**Figure 3–4**). In a *hordeolum*, the inflammation is caused by a staph bacterial infection, either on the inside or outside of the eyelid. An *internal hordeolum* occurs when the infection is in an oil gland inside the eye (a meibomian gland). An *external hordeolum* is when bacteria infect the root of an eyelash or one of the sweat glands. Antibiotics and anti-inflammatory drops can help treat a hordeolum.

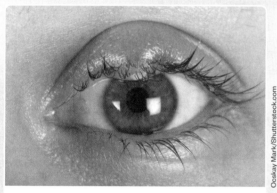

Fig. 3-4: Stye.

Chalazion

A **chalazion** is a swelling or lump on the eyelid that is caused by the buildup of materials within a meibomian gland (**Figure 3–5**). The gland becomes blocked and chronically infected, becoming a *granuloma*. The clear, oily material inside the gland becomes opaque and greasy. This is not a bacterial infection. Although it is less painful, it takes longer to resolve, and topical antibiotics don't work. Surgery may be an option.

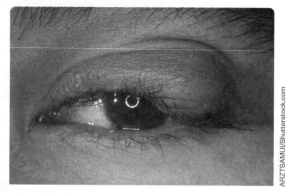

Fig. 3-5: Chalazion.

Ocular Rosacea

Ocular rosacea is an inflammation of the skin surrounding the eye, appearing as red, swollen, and highly sensitive eyelids or skin, possibly with broken blood vessels and acne-like bumps (**Figure 3–6**). Clients with ocular rosacea experience itchy, burning, dry eyes; blurred vision; makeup sensitivity; and acute light sensitivity. It is most common in adults with fair skin, hair, and eyes. Although this condition almost feels like pinkeye, ocular rosacea is not contagious. Chronic inflammation of the eyelid and hair follicles can cause premature hair loss. Clogged sebaceous glands along the margins of the eyelids and any discharge in the eye itself can be so hard that it damages the skin during removal.

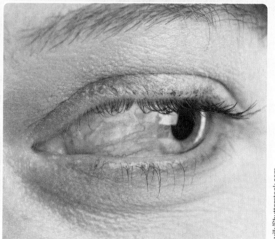

Fig. 3-6: Ocular rosacea.

Dry Eye Syndrome

Dry eye syndrome is the lack of proper tear production, either because the tear ducts fail to produce enough tears or the tears evaporate due to physical problems with the eye. Healthy tears have three layers; the eye can dry out if any of the layers are produced in the wrong amount. The oily outer layer keeps the tear from drying out. The salt water middle layer helps flush out foreign bodies. Without this, we produce a stringy substance from our eyelid glands, causing irritation. The mucous inner layer contains a protein that holds the layers of tears together and keeps them from sliding off the eye. Without this inner layer, the eye can more easily be overcome by allergies, conjunctivitis, or other disorders that cause the crusty sticking together of the eyes.

Contact Dermatitis

Dermatitis is a generalized term to refer to an inflammatory condition of the skin. **Contact dermatitis** is a skin inflammation caused by contact with certain chemicals or substances. There are two types of contact dermatitis: allergic contact dermatitis and irritant contact dermatitis. Dermatitis usually appears as a rash or itchy, dry skin, though skin eruptions are common. Wearing gloves or protective skin creams while working with chemicals or irritating substances can help prevent contact dermatitis. For eyelash clients, contact dermatitis can only occur where the skin is stimulated, for example, by placing extensions too close to the eyelid or due to irritation from adhesives, removers, or disinfectants.

ALLERGIC CONTACT DERMATITIS

Allergic contact dermatitis occurs when a person develops an allergy to an ingredient or a chemical, usually caused by repeated skin contact with the chemical. Once a product allergy is established, the person affected by the allergy (technician or client) must stop using that product until the allergic symptoms clear. In severe or chronic cases, affected people should see a dermatologist for allergy testing.

IRRITANT CONTACT DERMATITIS

Irritant contact dermatitis occurs when irritating substances temporarily damage the epidermis **(Figure 3-7)**. Unlike allergic contact dermatitis, irritant contact dermatitis is not usually chronic if precautions are taken. Adhesive removers and lash lifting solutions are examples of products with irritant potential. Contact with irritant chemicals can damage the epidermis because the irritant can enter the skin surface and cause inflammation, redness, swelling, itching, and burning. Repeated exposure can worsen the condition.

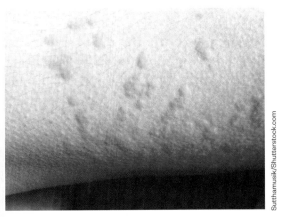

Fig. 3-7: Irritant contact dermatitis.

> **Did You Know?**
>
> Keeping your tools, equipment, and surfaces clean and disinfected is an important step in protecting yourself and avoiding skin problems. Practice these steps with great diligence:
>
> - Keep tools, containers, and tabletops clean and free from product, dust, and residue.
> - Wear protective gloves whenever using products known to cause irritant or allergic contact dermatitis.
> - Keep your hands clean and moisturized to prevent irritant reactions.

Ch. 03: Disorders, Diseases, and Allergies of the Eye Area

Ocular Herpes

Ocular herpes is an infection of the cornea, the retina, or the uvea (pigmented middle of the eye) caused by the herpes simplex virus. Severe cases can scar the cornea, causing visual impairment and even blindness. Ocular herpes presents as inflammation and redness, pain in one of the eyes, blurry vision, sensitivity to light, painful blisters, and even fever **(Figure 3–8)**. This condition is contagious.

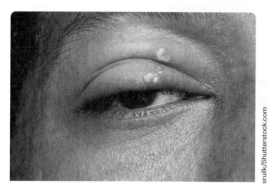

Fig. 3-8: Ocular herpes.

Seborrheic Dermatitis

Seborrheic dermatitis is a skin condition caused by chronic inflammation of the sebaceous glands and is often characterized by redness, dry or oily scaling, stubborn dandruff, crusting, and/or itchiness **(Figure 3–9)**. The red, flaky skin often appears in the eyebrows, beard, scalp, hairline, middle of the forehead, and sides of the nose. It is not contagious. The cause may be changes in skin cell functionality, environmental factors, an immune deficiency, or the colonization of lipophilic yeast.[1] Although seborrheic dermatitis is a medical condition, applying nonfatty skin care products designed for sensitive skin can help. Refer moderate to severe cases to a dermatologist.

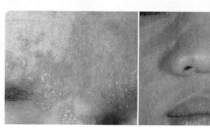

Fig. 3-9: Seborrheic dermatitis.

Eyelid and Lash Disorders

Additional eyelid and lash disorders can be found in **Table 3–1**.

Table 3-1		Eyelid and Lash Disorders
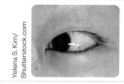	**Ectropion**	Causes the eyelid and lash to turn outward, usually the lower lids; involves loss of elasticity of the eyelid tissue and can require surgery to correct.
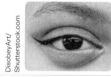	**Entropion**	Causes the eyelid to fold inward and the entire line of lashes to touch the cornea, which can scratch the cornea; involves loss of elasticity of the eyelid tissue and can require surgery to correct.
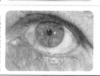	**Madarosis**	Loss of eyelashes or eyebrows, on one or both sides of the face.
	Trichiasis	Ingrowth of the lash, which can scratch the cornea.

Check In

2. What causes contact dermatitis?

   ....

   ....

3. What are demodex?

   ....

   ....

4. What part of the body does seborrheic dermatitis affect?

   ....

   ....

Workbook Assessment

Matching

For the following questions, match each statement to the correct letter choice.

QUESTION 1:

Match the eyelid and lash disorders with their descriptions.

............) a condition in which the eyelids droop outward

............) a condition in which the eyelids fold inward and the lashes touch the cornea

............) a condition in which a person loses the eyelashes or eyebrows on either or both sides of the face

............) a condition where the eyelashes grow toward the eye

Choices

A. madarosis
B. ectropion
C. trichiasis
D. entropion

Allergy Versus Sensitivity

> **Learning Objective 03**
>
> Identify allergies and sensitivities related to eyelash extensions.

The eyes are exposed to a constant stream of environmental allergens. The eyelashes do what they can by catching airborne dust, pollen, debris, mold, and pet dander, but innumerable irritants make it to the surface of the eyes and the surrounding skin. Although some allergies are seasonal, many are year-round and can make clients even more sensitive to adhesives and fumes. Itchy, swollen eyes are made worse when rubbing them causes microscopic cuts in eyelids, helping fumes and other irritants enter the body.

Sensitization

Although allergies are a natural reaction of the body to particular substances, an allergic reaction may not occur upon the first exposure. **Sensitization** is an allergic reaction created by *repeated* exposure to a chemical or a substance. Until the allergic reaction no longer occurs, the product causing the reaction must not be used. Eyelash adhesives and eyelash lift solutions can be common causes of allergic reactions with repeated exposure.

DOES IT GET BETTER OVER TIME?

Usually once you develop an allergic reaction it doesn't go away. Fortunately, hypersensitivity irritations are not permanent. If you avoid repeated and/or prolonged contact with the irritating substance, the skin will usually quickly repair itself; however, continued or repeated exposure may lead to chronic allergic reactions and skin damage.

Reasons for Reactions

Symptoms can develop over time or immediately. Many ingredients used in skin care products and treatments may cause adverse skin reactions. Fragrances and some preservatives and chemical sunscreen ingredients are among the most common allergens.

SYMPTOMS

It is often very difficult to distinguish whether a reaction is allergic or irritant. Physicians indicate that, in general, symptoms of an irritant reaction include burning, whereas itching is usually a sign of an allergic reaction. Additional symptoms may include inflammation of the skin, blisters, hives, or rashes. The eyes may swell, puff, or produce tears. In addition, adverse reactions may be detected immediately after product application, or may not show up until days or weeks later.

Being aware of a client's allergies and the ingredients being used in treatments is very important to avoid adverse reactions. During consultation, it's very important for a client to disclose any potential allergies. This should be indicated on their consultation form, and then verified again by the eyelash technician before proceeding with a treatment.

EYE PADS

The gel in eye pads can cause allergic reactions; always check the ingredients of pads being used. If you notice excessive tearing and redness with eye pads in place, consider that misuse rather than allergies/sensitivities may be the cause. Eye pads should never come in contact with the inside of the eye. Place pads 1 to 2 mm under the lash line, and never reuse eye pads.

If a pad is placed over the water line, under eye skin swelling can present as mild redness, tearing, burning sensation, or itching to a more severe inflammation. Eye pads can also cause bruised or bloodshot eyeballs or *corneal abrasion*—scraping or scratching of the cornea—and pain for a few days.

TAPES

Reactions to tape usually present as generalized redness, swelling, and bumpy, itchy skin of the whole eye area, not just along the upper lash line. To rule out a tape reaction, try using no stickers or tape on clients.

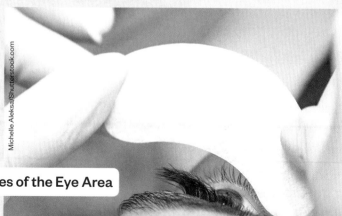

Michelle Aleksa/Shutterstock.com

ADHESIVES

Cyanoacrylate is the main ingredient in almost all adhesive, and a sensitivity to it may rule out eyelash application. Cyanoacrylate reactions can be difficult to distinguish from general irritation. An allergic reaction to cyanoacrylate shows up as a red, swollen, itchy lash line, or it can cause heavy swelling that closes the eyes shut. This reaction can occur even if the skin doesn't come into contact with adhesive.

- **Dyes.** Carbon black is a pigment or dye added to black lash glue to make it dark. Some people are allergic to carbon black; you may need to use an adhesive without it (usually clear).
- **Latex.** Latex adhesive reactions are similar to cyanoacrylate reactions, with itchy, red skin and possibly hives or rashes. Most clients will know if they have an allergy to latex and will likely tell you during the consultation. It is good practice to ask just in case.

IMPROPER ISOLATION

Improper isolation will cause lashes to not cycle through the full growing phase. This causes premature ripping out of the hair follicle, leading to itchiness, discomfort, and the client being unable to brush their lashes.

APPLICATION TOO CLOSE TO SKIN

Eyelash application too close to the skin can cause contact dermatitis, as glue is not meant to touch skin. A stye could also develop if an eyelash extension is able to touch the skin, causing irritation and red, inflamed, localized pain.

EYELASH LIFTING

Eyelash lifting can potentially cause blisters, rashes, and redness on the eyelid if the solution gets on the skin. Overprocessing the lashes is possible if the product is applied on the entire lash or left on past the processing time, which can lead to loss of lashes. Lash lifting can also cause irritation and damage of the eye if contacted by the lifting solution.

EYELASH AND EYEBROW TINTING

Blisters, rashes, watery eyes, inflammation, and weak lashes can result from eyelash and eyebrow tinting. Contact dermatitis can occur if the tinting solution touches the skin, and the fumes given off from the service can irritate the eye without contacting it. Bear in mind that lash and brow tinting are outside of an eyelash technician or esthetician's scope of service in some states.

EYEBROW LAMINATION

The solution used for eyebrow lamination can also cause redness, swelling, itching, and bumps if it contacts the skin around the brows. As with other eyelash and eyebrow services, careful application—combined with patch tests—is key.

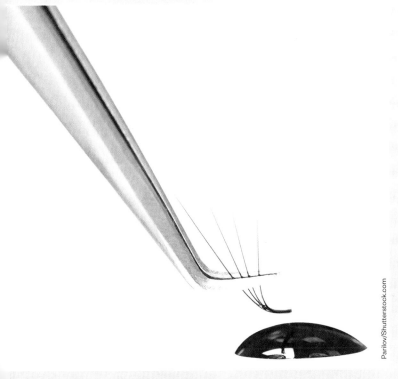

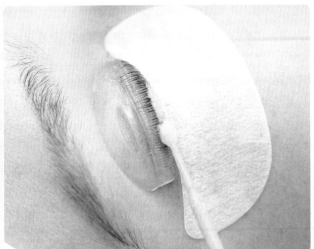

Ch. 03: Disorders, Diseases, and Allergies of the Eye Area

Patch Tests

If you or the client have concerns about reactions, schedule a patch test 48 hours or more before a service. If there is any reaction within 24 hours, do not use the product. Find a replacement (and test again) or cancel the service.

- Adhesive—Apply 4 to 8 lashes per eye, dispersed evenly through the lashes, contacting only the eyelash follicle and avoiding any contact with the skin, and wait 24 hours **(Figure 3–10)**. If the client feels any sensation, or if the skin becomes itchy, irritated, or red, remove the test lashes, preferably using the banana peel technique.

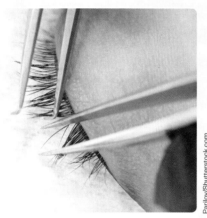

Fig. 3-10: Apply a few lashes to determine if a client is allergic to any products 48 hours before a service.

- Lifting—Apply the product to the nape of the neck, behind the ear, or to the side of the arm and wait 24 hours.
- Tinting—Apply the product to the nape of the neck, behind the ear, or to the side of the arm and wait 24 hours.
- Tape—Apply the product behind the ear or to the side of the arm and wait 24 hours.
- Eye pads—Apply the product behind the ear or to the side of the arm and wait 24 hours.

HOW TO HANDLE AN ADVERSE REACTION

If a client complains of burning or their skin becomes excessively irritated during a procedure, immediately remove the product, rinse the area with cold water, and apply cool compresses. It is recommended for salons and studios to have products that calm skin reactions as a precaution. If adhesive or chemicals touch the eye, if the eye begins watering, or if the client complains of stinging or burning, immediately flush the eye(s) using an eyewash station or kit, and tell the client to seek help from a medical professional.

 Caution!

Keep original packaging and labeling from the product manufacturer for a full list of all of the specific ingredients to prevent allergic or adverse reaction to a product.

 Check In

5. How does hypersensitivity differ from an allergy?

6. How long should you wait for a patch test to process? How long before a service should you administer a patch test?

7. What should a technician do if during a treatment the client has an adverse reaction?

Workbook Assessment

Please circle the correct answer for each question below.

Multiple Choice

QUESTION 2:

In the context of allergy and sensitivity, which of the following statements are true of an allergic reaction?

A) An allergic reaction to a chemical may develop on repeated exposure to the chemical.

B) If an allergic reaction does not occur at the first exposure to an allergen, it is unlikely to occur in the future.

C) Once an allergic reaction subsides, the chemical that caused the reaction can usually be safely used again.

D) Once an allergic reaction develops, it usually does not go away.

QUESTION 3:

Which of the following should you keep in mind while using eye pads during a lash service?

A) The gel in eye pads is hypoallergenic and not likely to cause allergic reactions.

B) Eye pads should never touch the inside of the eye.

C) Eye pads must never be reused.

D) Eye pads must never be placed within 10 mm of the lash line.

QUESTION 4:

Which of the following are true of cyanoacrylate?

A) It is used in most of the lash adhesives.

B) Its reactions can be easily distinguished from those of general irritation.

C) It can cause an allergic reaction even if it does not directly touch the skin.

D) Allergic reactions are very mild and painless.

QUESTION 5:

Which of the following is likely to occur if a lash technician fails to isolate the lashes properly during the application of lash extensions?

A) The client will be unable to brush the extensions.

B) The growth phase of natural lashes will be disrupted.

C) The hair follicles may be pulled out prematurely.

D) The client will get symptoms of contact dermatitis.

QUESTION 6:

Which of the following actions can cause overprocessing of the lashes while performing an eyelash lift?

A) applying the product on the entire lash

B) touching the product to the skin of the eyelid

C) leaving on the product for more time than is required for processing

D) touching the product to the inner eye

QUESTION 7:

Identify the potential adverse reaction(s) that can occur from using eyelash and eyebrow tinting solution.

A) It can cause dry eye syndrome.

B) It can cause contact dermatitis if it comes into contact with the skin.

C) Its fumes can irritate the eyes without touching the eyes.

D) It can cause the lashes to weaken.

QUESTION 8:

Imagine you are applying lash extensions to a client and the adhesive accidentally touches the client's eye. Which of the following should you do?

A) Use an eyewash kit to immediately flush the eye.

B) Apply a warm compress.

C) Tell the client to visit a medical professional.

D) Use a solvent to quickly remove the adhesive from the eye.

Chapter Glossary

allergic contact dermatitis *uh-**LUR**-jihk **KAHN**-takt der-muh-**TAI**-tis*	p. 039	an allergy to an ingredient or a chemical, usually caused by repeated skin contact with the chemical
blepharitis *bleh-fuh-**RYE**-tis*	p. 037	inflammation of the eyelids; chronically difficult to treat and causes dry eyes with occasional crusting or flakey material on the eyelashes after sleeping; commonly caused by staphylococcus
chalazion *kuh-**LAY**-zee-uhn*	p. 038	swelling or lump on the eyelid that is caused by the buildup of materials within a meibomian gland
conjunctivitis *kuhn-juhngk-tuh-**VAI**-tis*	p. 037	also known as *pinkeye*; eye infection that may be caused by bacteria or virus; can be extremely contagious

Term	Page	Definition
contact dermatitis *KAHN-takt der-mah-**TAI**-tis*	p. 039	skin inflammation caused by contact with certain chemicals or substances
demodex ***DEH**-muh-deks*	p. 038	contagious condition where microscopic mites burrow into and live inside the eyelash hair follicle; eyelash hair loss and potentially blindness
dry eye syndrome *drai ai **SIN**-drohm*	p. 039	lack of proper tear production, either because the tear ducts fail to produce enough tears or the tears evaporate due to physical problems with the eye
ectropion *ek-**TROH**-pee-ahn*	p. 040	causes the eyelid and lash to turn outward, usually the lower lids; involves loss of elasticity of the eyelid tissue and can require surgery to correct
entropion *uhn-**TROH**-pee-ahn*	p. 040	causes the eyelid to fold inward and the entire line of lashes to touch the cornea, which can scratch the cornea; involves loss of elasticity of the eyelid tissue and can require surgery to correct
madarosis *muh-duh-**ROH**-sis*	p. 040	loss of eyelashes or eyebrows, on one or both sides of the face
ocular herpes ***AH**-kyuh-lur **HER**-peez*	p. 040	contagious infection of the cornea, the retina, or the uvea caused by the herpes simplex virus
ocular rosacea ***AH**-kyuh-lur row-**ZAY**-shuh*	p. 038	inflammation of the skin surrounding the eye, appearing as red, swollen, and highly sensitive eyelids or skin, possibly with broken blood vessels and acne-like bumps
seborrheic dermatitis *seb-oh-**REE**-ick der-mah-**TAI**-tis*	p. 040	skin condition caused by chronic inflammation of the sebaceous glands; often characterized by redness, dry or oily scaling, crusting, stubborn dandruff, and/or itchiness
sensitization *sen-sih-ti-**ZAY**-shun*	p. 042	allergic reaction created by repeated exposure to a chemical or a substance
stye *sty*	p. 038	inflammation of a Zeis or meibomian gland that appears as a painful, red bump on the eyelid
trichiasis *try-**KY**-uh-sis*	p. 040	ingrowth of the lash, which can scratch the cornea

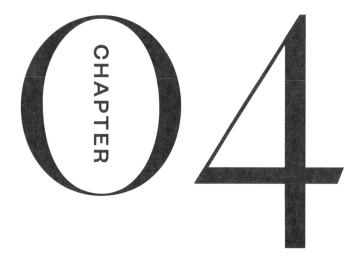

CHAPTER 04

Client Safety and Infection Control

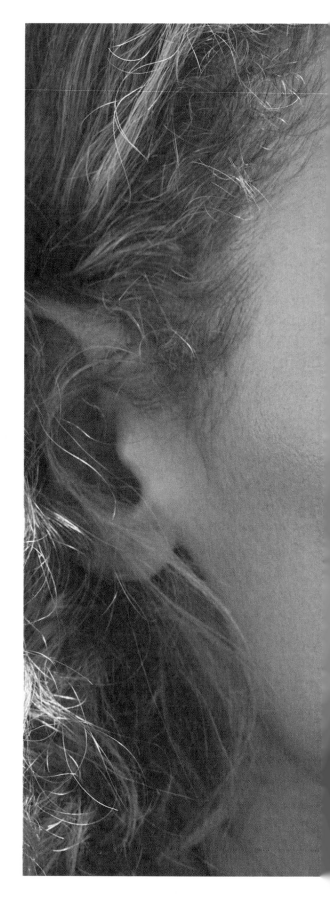

🚩 **Learning Objectives**

After completing this chapter, you will be able to:

1. Explain why eyelash technicians need to understand client safety and infection control.
2. Review the basics of infection control.
3. Employ proper hand washing technique.
4. Demonstrate effective disinfection of tools and work surfaces.
5. Follow exposure protocols to protect yourself and your clients.

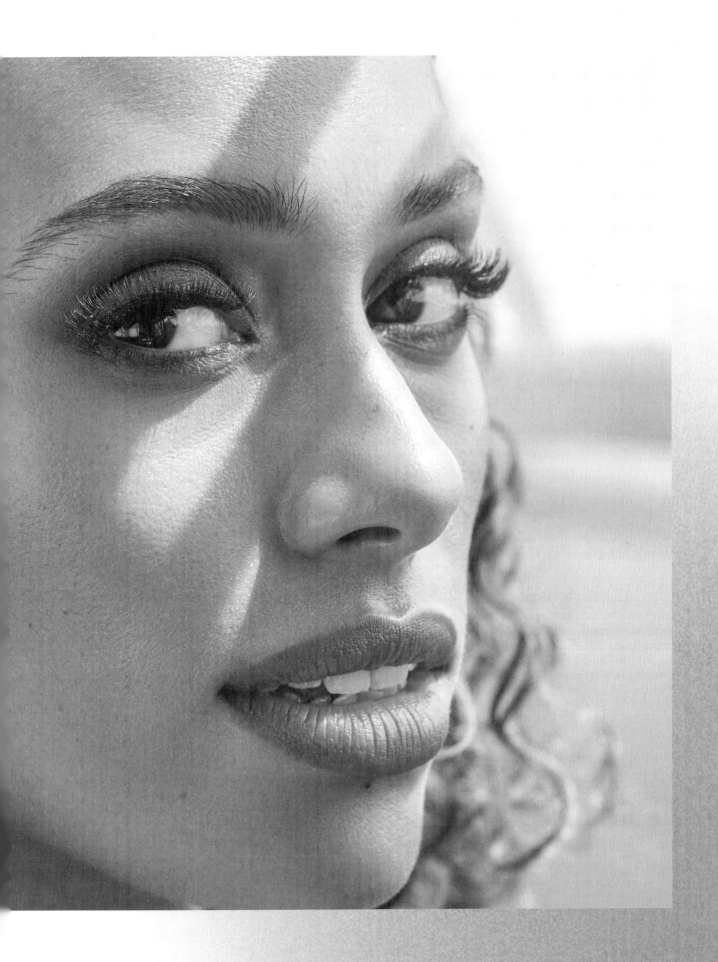

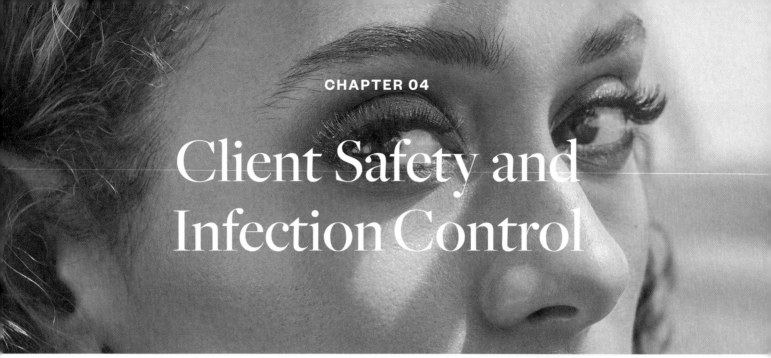

CHAPTER 04

Client Safety and Infection Control

Why Study Client Safety and Infection Control?

 Learning Objective 01

Explain why eyelash technicians need to understand client safety and infection control.

Having a thorough understanding of infection control principles and practices is necessary when dealing with the public and coming into daily direct contact with clients. Practicing the basics of cleaning and disinfecting and following federal and state rules will safeguard your health as well as the health of your clients.

Eyelash technicians should study and have a thorough understanding of client safety and infection control because:

- As an eyelash technician you will have daily contact with your client's skin and eyes, both important avenues of infection.
- Knowledge of products and practices to prevent the spread of infection will ensure a safe work environment for the technician and the client.
- You must understand and practice techniques to prevent and control exposure to not only blood but also other potentially infectious material to protect your health and the health of your clients.

 Check In

1. Why do you think it is important to study client safety and infection control?

Infection Control Basics

 Learning Objective 02

Review the basics of infection control.

It is your responsibility as an eyelash technician to use proper and effective infection control methods that help safeguard your health and the health of your clients. You are also responsible for employing safe work practices to help prevent accidents and injuries from occurring in the workplace.

The standard for hygiene is the protocol followed by dentist offices. Treat every client as if they are harboring harmful microbes. Prevent cross-contamination by always using cleaned and disinfected products, tools, and work surfaces. Immediately discard single-use products, and consider all hands, tools, products, and surfaces contaminated as soon as they are touched to a human body.

Prevention 101

In general, the risk of infection can be greatly reduced with a few simple steps:

- Eliminate pathogens through proper hand washing, cleaning, and disinfection or sterilization.
- Clean and disinfect tools and equipment after every service.
- Keep your skin intact to reduce portals of entry for bacteria. Wear gloves when working with chemicals, use lotion to reduce skin drying and cracking, and cover open wounds.
- Be prepared to turn away or reschedule clients who show signs of illness. Remember, you are not licensed to diagnose illness or infection. Refer sick patients to their healthcare provider for a proper diagnosis and treatment regimen.

Personal Habits

It is important to think about your personal habits in terms of how they might increase or decrease the risk of transmitting an illness. For example, if you see 50 clients a week and you shake hands with each of them, you are exposing yourself to everything on the hands of those 50 people every week—it could be only a matter of time before you get sick! However, making a habit of following the rules of proper cleaning and disinfection, both in your home and at work, will help decrease the odds of falling ill. Hand washing, cleaning, and disinfection are all ways in which you can personally combat the spread of disease and safeguard your health and that of your clients.

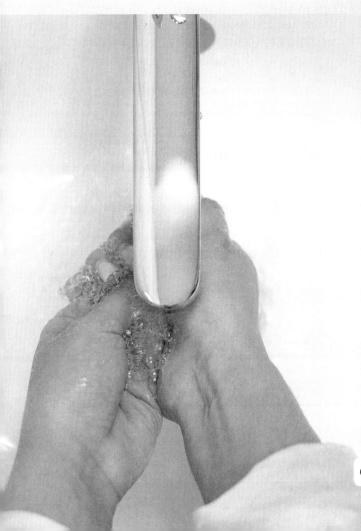

Edward Jenner/Pexels.com

 Check In

2. How can you greatly reduce the risk of infection on the job?

Ch. 04: Client Safety and Infection Control

Workbook Assessment

Please circle the correct answer for each question below.

Multiple Choice

QUESTION 1:
Which of the following should eyelash technicians do to ensure a high level of infection control?

A) Clean work surfaces twice every day, before the first client and after the last client.

B) Sterilize masks and gloves after every use.

C) Ask the clients to fill out an intake form.

D) Assume that every client is carrying harmful pathogens.

QUESTION 2:
How can lash technicians prevent cross-contamination?

A) by avoiding the use of single-use products

B) by using cleaned and disinfected products, tools, and work surfaces

C) by completing patch tests for all products before starting a service

D) by insisting that clients bring a doctor's note to every appointment

QUESTION 3:
To control the spread of infectious diseases, the ideal hygiene protocol for lash salons is the protocol followed where?

A) at home

B) at family clinics

C) at dentists' offices

D) at restaurants

QUESTION 4:
Identify the correct statement about when a tool may be considered to be contaminated.

A) A tool is considered contaminated even if it comes into contact with intact human skin.

B) A tool is considered contaminated if it comes into contact with any body fluid but not when it comes into contact with intact human skin.

C) A tool is not considered contaminated if it comes into contact with human skin, even if the skin is broken.

D) A tool is not considered contaminated if it comes into contact with saliva but is considered contaminated if it comes into contact with blood.

Ch. 04: Client Safety and Infection Control

QUESTION 5:

Which of the following steps must a lash technician follow to reduce the risk of infection?

    A) Exclusively use antibacterial soaps.

    B) Avoid hand lotions.

    C) Use petroleum-based gloves when working with petroleum-based products.

    D) Eliminate pathogens with proper hand washing.

QUESTION 6:

One of your regular clients comes in for a lash refill service. When you talk to the client, they mention having a cold. The client says they really need a lash refill as they are leaving for a business trip soon. Which of the following should you do?

    A) Reschedule for when the client is well or has been cleared by a healthcare provider.

    B) Provide the service as usual as you believe the client that it is just a seasonal allergy.

    C) Provide the lash refill service to the client in an isolated area to protect others.

    D) Conduct a proper diagnosis to rule out cold or flu and then decide whether to provide the service.

Hand Washing

 Learning Objective 03

Employ proper hand washing technique.

Properly washing your hands is one of the most important actions you can take to prevent spreading germs from one person to another. Proper hand washing removes germs from the folds and grooves of the skin and from under the free edge of the nail plate by lifting and rinsing germs and contaminants from the surface of your skin. You should wash your hands thoroughly before and after working with each client. Follow the hand washing procedure described in **Procedure 4–1: Proper Hand Washing**.

 Perform:

Perform 4-1: Proper Hand Washing

 Caution!

When washing hands, use liquid soaps in pump or automatic dispensing containers. Bacteria can grow in bar soaps.

Ch. 04: Client Safety and Infection Control

Antibacterial Soaps

Although there are many marketing claims on soaps these days, antibacterial and antimicrobial soaps have been under Food and Drug Administration (FDA) scrutiny since 2014. In 2016, many of the chemicals used in these soaps were banned. What's more, research has shown that repeated use of antibacterial products can increase the growth of some of the worst pathogens. The true benefit of hand washing comes from the friction created by the soap bubbles that works to "pull" pathogens off the skin surface. Repeated hand washing can also dry the skin, so using a moisturizing hand lotion after washing is a good practice. Be sure the hand lotion is in a pump container, not a jar.

Avoid using very hot water to wash your hands because this is another practice that can damage the skin. Remember, you must wash your hands thoroughly before and after each service, so do all you can to reduce any irritation that may occur.

Waterless Hand Sanitizers

Hand sanitizers generally contain a high volume of alcohol and are intended to reduce the numbers and slow the growth of microbes on the skin **(Figure 4–1)**. When there is visible dirt/debris on the hands, neither waterless hand sanitizers nor antiseptics will work until the dirt/debris is removed; this can be accomplished only with liquid soap, a soft-bristle brush, and water.

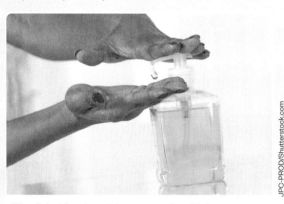

Fig. 4-1: Hand sanitizers contain a high concentration of alcohol.

Due to the drying effect of alcohol, hand sanitizers should not be overused, but, if allowed by your state, they are an excellent option when hand washing is not possible. Never use an antiseptic to disinfect instruments or other surfaces. It is ineffective for that purpose. Be aware that the high percentage of alcohol can dry the skin to the point of causing openings that allow for infectious agents to infect you. With that in mind, use hand sanitizers only as a secondary option to hand washing.

 Check In

3. What is a side effect of both repeated hand washing and hand sanitizer overuse that should be counteracted to maintain skin health?

Workbook Assessment

Select whether the statements below are true or false.

True or False

QUESTION 7:

Rahim, who has recently joined an eyelash technician training program, thinks that technicians need to wash their hands with soap before and after every service only if they are not planning to wear gloves during the service. In the given scenario, Rahim is correct in their assumption.

T F why?..

QUESTION 8:

Eyelash technicians must avoid using bar soaps and instead use liquid soap in a pump container to wash their hands.

T F why?..

QUESTION 9:

When washing hands, you must use the fingernails of one hand to remove any visible debris from under the fingernails of the other hand.

T F why?..

QUESTION 10:

When washing hands, after using the nail brush, you must immediately rinse the soap out of it and keep it on a paper towel to dry so that it is ready for the next appointment.

T F why?..

QUESTION 11:

After washing your hands for an eyelash service, you must avoid touching the faucet or doorknobs with bare fingers.

T F why?..

QUESTION 12:

Research shows that repeated use of antibacterial products in soaps can increase the growth of some of the harmful bacteria.

T F why?..

QUESTION 13:

Hand sanitizers are more effective than liquid soap and water in removing dirt and debris from hands.

T F why?..

QUESTION 14:

Alcohol-based sanitizers work by slowing down the growth of microbes on the skin of the hands.

T F why?..

QUESTION 15:

Your current appointment of lash extension application service runs longer than anticipated, and you are late for your next appointment. To save time, you decide to spray your tools with an antiseptic spray and wipe them instead of following the complete procedure of washing and disinfecting tools. In the given scenario, it is acceptable for you to use your tools for your next appointment.

T F why?..

Cleaning and Disinfecting

 Learning Objective 04

Demonstrate effective disinfection of tools and work surfaces.

Proper infection control can prevent the spread of disease caused by exposure to potentially infectious materials on an item's surface. Infection control will also prevent exposure to blood and visible debris or residue such as dust, hair, and skin.

Use Environmental Protection Agency (EPA)-approved disinfectants on surfaces and tools, although autoclaves and flash sterilizers are acceptable for multiuse implements. Cleanse doorknobs, counters, and treatment beds or chairs to prevent the spread of common eye disease. Practice proper infection control habits and a work area preparation routine for each client.

Cleaning and Disinfecting Nonporous, Reusable Items

State rules require that all multiuse tools and implements be cleaned and disinfected before every service. Mix all disinfectants according to the manufacturer's directions, always adding the disinfectant to the water rather than the water to the disinfectant **(Figure 4–2)**. Follow the cleaning and disinfecting nonporous, reusable items procedure described in **Procedure 4–2: Cleaning and Disinfecting Nonporous, Reusable Items**.

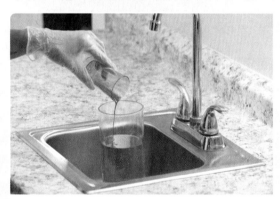

Fig. 4-2: Carefully pour the disinfectant into the water when preparing disinfectant solution.

PROPER USE OF DISINFECTANTS

Implements must be thoroughly cleaned of all visible matter or residue before being placed in disinfectant solution. This is because residue will interfere with the disinfectant and prevent proper disinfection. Properly cleaned implements and tools, free from all visible debris, must be completely immersed in disinfectant solution. *Complete immersion* means there is enough liquid in the container to cover all surfaces of the item being disinfected, including the handles, for 10 minutes or for the time recommended by the manufacturer **(Figure 4–3)**. When using a spray, wipe, or aerosol disinfectant, you must still look for and adhere to the contact time to ensure that all pathogens on the label are being effectively destroyed. *Sprays* are used for larger tools and implements that cannot or should not be immersed. *Wipes* are used for surfaces and other nonsubmersible items.

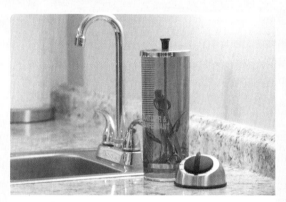

Fig. 4-3: Implements must be completely immersed in disinfectant solution.

Perform:

Perform 4-2: Cleaning and Disinfecting Nonporous, Reusable Items

Sterilizers

Sterilization, the process that destroys all microbial life, including spores, can be incorporated into cleaning routines but is rarely mandated. Effective sterilization typically requires the use of an autoclave or flash sterilizer **(Figure 4–4)**—equipment that applies both heat and pressure. For sterilization to be effective, items must be cleaned prior to use and the sterilizer must be tested and maintained as instructed in the manufacturer's specifications. The Centers for Disease Control and Prevention (CDC) requires that autoclaves and sterilizers be tested monthly to ensure they are properly sterilizing implements. The accepted method is called a *spore test*. Sealed packages containing test organisms are subjected to a typical sterilization cycle and then sent to a contract laboratory that specializes in sterilizer performance testing.

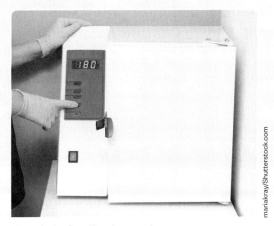

Fig. 4-4: Sterilization equipment.

 Caution!

Although they can make effective storage options after disinfection or sterilization, UV light units do not effectively sterilize implements.

Disinfecting Equipment

Electrical equipment has contact points that cannot be completely immersed in liquid. These items should be cleaned and disinfected using an EPA-registered disinfectant designed for use on these devices. Follow the procedures recommended by the disinfectant manufacturer for preparing the solution and follow the item's manufacturer directions for cleaning and disinfecting the device.

Disinfecting Work Surfaces

Most states require that all work surfaces be cleaned and disinfected before beginning a service. Be sure to clean and disinfect tables, stations, chairs, armrests, and any other surface that a customer's skin may have touched. Clean doorknobs and handles daily to reduce transfer of germs to your hands.

Cleaning Towels and Linens

Clean towels and linens should be used for each client. To clean towels, linens, and capes, launder according to the directions on the item's label. Be sure that towels and linens are thoroughly dried. Items that are not dry may grow mildew and bacteria. Store soiled linens and towels in covered or closed containers, away from clean linens and towels, even if your state regulatory agency does not require that you do so. Whenever possible, use disposable towels, especially in restrooms.

Multiuse Products

When using creams, lotions, gels, or any other product that is dispensed from a multiuse container, it is important not to contaminate the product. Always use a pump or shaker to dispense products when possible. For products in a tub-type container, always use a clean spatula (disposable or disinfectable) to remove the product—never use your fingers!

APPROPRIATE HANDLING OF SINGLE-USE ITEMS

- Soiled items such as gloves and under-eye pads must be placed in a covered waste container.
- While in use, single-use items must be placed on surfaces that can be disinfected or disposed of, such as a paper towel.
- Keep clean supplies separate from used ones. Take out only what is needed for each service **(Figure 4–5)**.

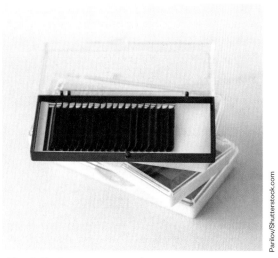

Fig. 4-5: Remove strips of eyelash extensions from their containers for each service.

 Caution!

Any sharp single-use instruments used in your workplace—such as needles or razors—should go in a sharps disposal container. These are hard red, yellow, or clear plastic containers marked with a biohazard symbol and governed by specific handling instructions.

Properly Clean and Disinfect the Treatment Area

The pre-service procedure is an organized, step-by-step plan for cleaning and disinfecting your implements, assembling materials, organizing your station, and meeting your client. Refer to **Procedure 4–3: Pre-Service Procedure** for the complete steps.

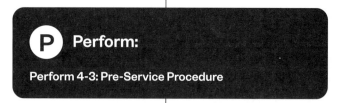

Perform:

Perform 4-3: Pre-Service Procedure

The post-service procedure is an organized, step-by-step plan for caring for your client after the procedure has been completed, as well as cleaning the treatment area at the end of the service and the end of the day. It details how to help your client through the scheduling and payment process and allows you to close the service by offering rebooking dates and retail home care purchases. Refer to **Procedure 4–4: Post-Service Procedure** for the complete steps.

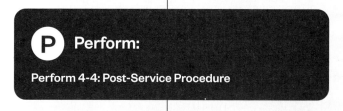

Perform:

Perform 4-4: Post-Service Procedure

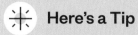 **Here's a Tip**

Facility guidelines for cleaning up will vary, especially as infection control procedures improve as laws and technology evolve. Be aware of regional laws and regulations.

Disinfectant Tips and Safety

Never forget that disinfectants are poisonous and can cause serious skin and eye damage. Some disinfectants appear clear, whereas others, especially phenolic disinfectants, are a little cloudy. Always use caution when handling disinfectants, in addition to using the tips below.

Always

- Keep the Safety Data Sheet (SDS) on hand for the disinfectant(s) you use.
- Wear gloves and safety glasses **(Figure 4-6)**.

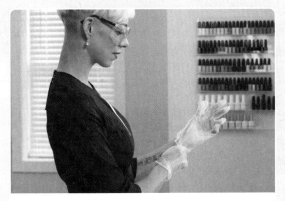

Fig. 4-6: Wear gloves and safety glasses while handling disinfectants.

- Avoid skin and eye contact.
- Add disinfectant to water when diluting (rather than adding water to a disinfectant) to prevent foaming, which can result in an incorrect mixing ratio.
- Use tongs, gloves, or a draining basket to remove implements from disinfectants.
- Keep disinfectants out of reach of children.
- Follow the manufacturer's instructions for mixing, using, and disposing of disinfectants.
- Use disinfectants only on clean hard, nonporous surfaces.
- Keep an item submerged in the disinfectant for 10 minutes unless the product label specifies differently.
- Immerse the entire implement in disinfectant if the product label calls for "complete immersion."
- To disinfect large surfaces, such as countertops, carefully apply the disinfectant to the clean surface or use a disinfectant spray and allow it to remain moist for 10 minutes, unless state regulations say differently.
- Strictly follow the manufacturer's directions for when to replace the disinfectant solution in order to ensure the healthiest conditions for you and your client. Replace the disinfectant solution every day—more often if the solution becomes soiled or contaminated.
- Wear gloves for all procedures to prevent contamination and protect hands from strong chemicals. Wash hands after completing infection control procedures.
- To avoid cross-contamination, roll the used side of linens and sheets inward so the dirty side is inside the laundry bundle. This also helps keep product and hair off the floor and saves cleaning time. For additional cleanliness, do not let linens or other items touch your clothing before or after use.
- Disinfect any magnifying lamps.
- If you use a towel warmer, turn it off and disinfect the bottom tray and the inside of the machine after removing all used items.
- Disinfect any other equipment that was used and turn it off.
- Clean all containers and wipe off dirty product containers with a disinfectant.
- Clean all counters, sinks, surfaces, and floor mats with disinfectant.

Never

- Let quats, phenols, bleach, or any other disinfectant come in contact with your skin. If you do get disinfectant on your skin, immediately wash the area with liquid soap and warm water. Then, rinse and dry the area thoroughly.
- Place any disinfectant or other product in an unmarked container. All containers should be labeled with, at the least, the product name, ingredients, date of mixing, and manufacturer's information.
- Mix chemicals together unless specified in the manufacturer's instructions. (For example, mixing bleach and ammonia products or bleach and vinegar creates potentially fatal toxic vapors!)

In addition, make sure to change the disinfectant to comply with the manufacturer's directions and infection control regulations. If required, record on a dated log when the disinfectant is changed **(Table 4–1)**.

Table 4-1   Example Disinfectant Log

DISINFECTANT LOG

Change the disinfectant solution in the container according to the manufacturer's directions or if it is cloudy and seems to require changing. Record when it is changed.

DATE CHANGED	YOUR INITIALS
March 5th	J.S.

Caution!

Improper mixing of disinfectants—to be weaker or more concentrated than the manufacturer's instructions—can significantly reduce their effectiveness. Always add the disinfectant concentrate to the water when mixing, and always follow the manufacturer's instructions for proper dilution.

Safety glasses and gloves should be worn while mixing to avoid accidental contact with eyes and skin.

Safety Data Sheets

The Occupational Safety and Health Administration (OSHA) Hazard Communication Standard requires that employees be notified of any chemical in their workplace that could be hazardous. Prior to 2015, the Material Safety Data Sheet (MSDS) was the document used to provide this information to workers and first responders. In 2015, these were replaced by the **Safety Data Sheet (SDS)**. Although both sheets provide essentially the same important information about chemicals, the organization and ease of understanding has been greatly improved in the SDS.

All SDSs are formatted into 16 categories, with nine accepted pictograms, and are provided for free from the manufacturer of the chemical. Having an SDS available for every chemical used in the workplace is a requirement of OSHA. In addition,, SDSs must be immediately available to all employees, so storing them on a computer that only managers can access or keeping them in a locked office is not acceptable **(Figure 4–7)**. Remember, these sheets are for use in emergencies, which are often chaotic situations where every second counts.

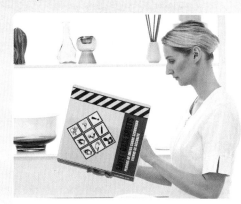

Fig. 4-7: Safety Data Sheets must be immediately available to all employees in the event of an emergency.

SDS CATEGORIES

The categories on the SDS are in a uniform format and order that must be followed by all manufacturers:

1. Identification. Includes the name of the product and contact information for the manufacturer or distributor; also contains recommended use and restrictions on use
2. Hazard(s) Identification. Lists all hazards associated with the product and includes hazard classification (flammable, etc.), precautionary statements, and hazard pictograms **(Figure 4–8)**

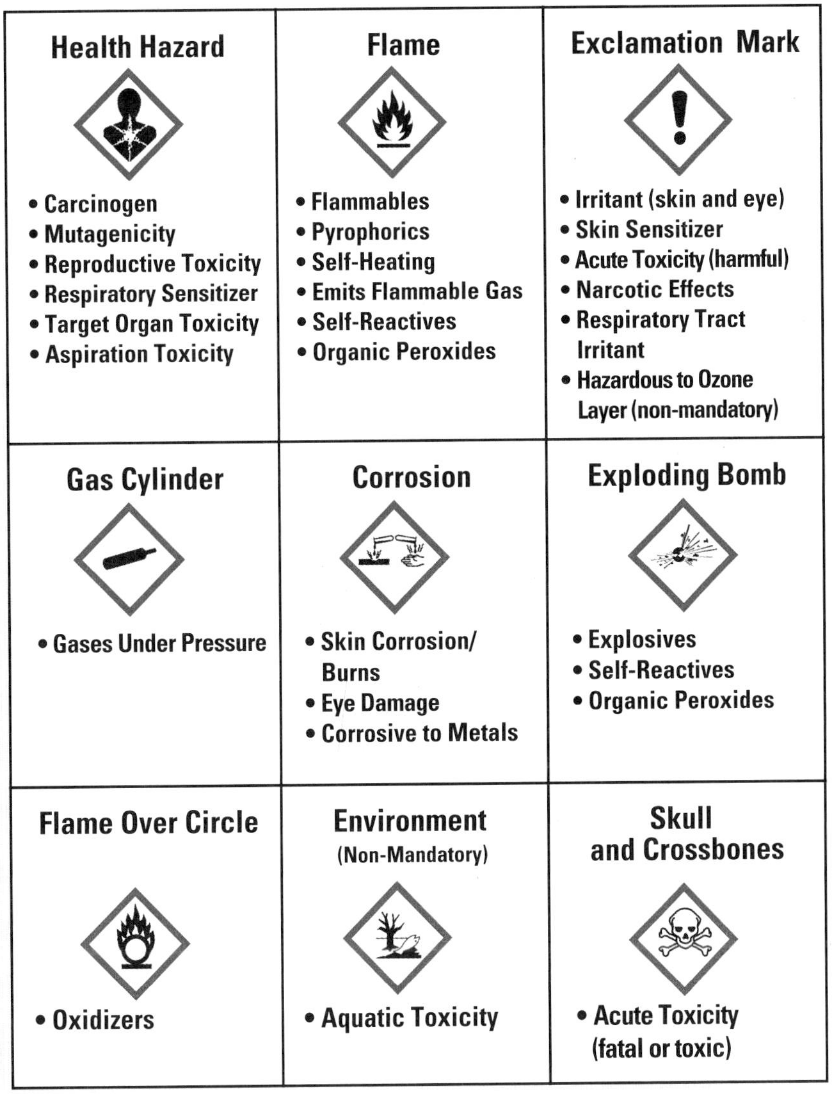

Health Hazard	Flame	Exclamation Mark
• Carcinogen • Mutagenicity • Reproductive Toxicity • Respiratory Sensitizer • Target Organ Toxicity • Aspiration Toxicity	• Flammables • Pyrophorics • Self-Heating • Emits Flammable Gas • Self-Reactives • Organic Peroxides	• Irritant (skin and eye) • Skin Sensitizer • Acute Toxicity (harmful) • Narcotic Effects • Respiratory Tract Irritant • Hazardous to Ozone Layer (non-mandatory)
Gas Cylinder	**Corrosion**	**Exploding Bomb**
• Gases Under Pressure	• Skin Corrosion/Burns • Eye Damage • Corrosive to Metals	• Explosives • Self-Reactives • Organic Peroxides
Flame Over Circle	**Environment** (Non-Mandatory)	**Skull and Crossbones**
• Oxidizers	• Aquatic Toxicity	• Acute Toxicity (fatal or toxic)

Fig. 4-8: Safety Data Sheet hazard pictograms dictated by the international Globally Harmonized System of Classification and Labelling of Chemicals (GHS).

Ch. 04: Client Safety and Infection Control

3. Composition/Information on Ingredients. Identifies the ingredients in the product, including concentrations used in mixtures and when chemical names have been withheld due to a trade secret

4. First-Aid Measures. Includes short- and long-term symptoms and first-aid instructions

5. Fire-Fighting Measures. Lists suitable (and unsuitable) fire extinguishers, any chemical hazards associated with a fire, and recommended protective equipment or precautions

6. Accidental Release Measures. Provides instruction for proper cleanup of a spill, protective equipment needed, and emergency measures to follow

7. Handling and Storage. Includes guidelines for safe handling and storage of chemicals, including incompatible chemicals

8. Exposure Controls/Personal Protection. Provides recommended limits on exposure and methods to reduce exposure, such as personal protective equipment (PPE) and proper ventilation

9. Physical and Chemical Properties. Consists of a minimum of 18 properties, from color to pH to viscosity; unknown or irrelevant properties for a product must be noted

10. Stability and Reactivity. Provides information on the environmental, stability, and reaction risks associated with the product

11. Toxicological Information. Details the risks of exposure, including symptoms such as skin irritation, and measure of toxicity

12. Ecological Information. Covers the impact of the chemical on the environment, such as groundwater absorption or danger to plants and animals

13. Disposal Considerations. Lists any procedures for disposal

14. Transport Information. Provides guidelines and restrictions for safe transportation

15. Regulatory Information. Includes any specific safety, health, or environmental regulations

16. Other Information. Indicates when the SDS was created or last updated[1]

SDS VOCABULARY

SDSs make use of a wide range of scientific, medical, and specialized vocabulary to describe chemical properties and hazards. Although it is well beyond the scope of this text to tackle SDS vocabulary, it is important to make a distinction between two pairs of related terms:

- A *carcinogen* is a substance that causes or is believed to cause cancer. A *mutagen*, on the other hand, is a substance that may cause cancer but not always. Mutagens cause an increase in cellular mutations (changes), some of which are harmful; others have little or no effect on the body's function.

- *Combustible* material is capable of igniting and burning. Compared to this, flammable (FLA-ma-bul) material is even easier to ignite—combustible liquid has a flashpoint between 100 and 200 degrees Fahrenheit, whereas flammable liquid has a flashpoint below 100 degrees. The term "inflammable" is an older term, meaning flammable; nonflammable signifies something is not flammable.

 Check In

4. How long should an item be fully submerged in disinfectant?

5. What is the difference between disinfecting and sterilizing?

6. Where should SDSs be stored?

Workbook Assessment

Matching

For the following questions, match each statement to the correct letter choice.

QUESTION 16:

Match the categories on the Safety Data Sheet (SDS) of a chemical to the information that is provided in that category about the chemical.

............) recommended uses and restrictions on use

............) concentrations used in mixtures

............) incompatibility with other chemicals

............) the pH of the chemical

............) problems associated with groundwater absorption

Choices

A. Handling and Storage
B. Identification
C. Composition/Information on Ingredients
D. Ecological Information
E. Physical and Chemical Properties

QUESTION 17:

Match the categories on the Safety Data Sheet (SDS) of a chemical that contains information about the recommended action to the described scenarios.

............) if you spill the disinfectant while preparing the disinfectant solution

............) if your colleague splashes themselves with a chemical and experiences a burning sensation

............) if you want to know if it is all right to keep the chemical in a room with direct sunlight

............) if you want to know where to discard used chemicals

Choices

A. First-Aid Measures
B. Accidental Release Measures
C. Disposal Considerations
D. Handling and Storage

Ch. 04: Client Safety and Infection Control

Exposure Incidents

Learning Objective 05

Follow exposure protocols to protect yourself and your clients.

Standard Precautions (SP) are guidelines published by the CDC that require the employer and employee to assume that any human blood and other body fluids are potentially infectious. Because it may not be possible to identify clients with infectious diseases, and such clients may not look sick, strict infection control practices should be used with all clients. In many instances, clients may be just getting sick or may be long-term viral carriers and are **asymptomatic**, meaning that they show no symptoms or signs of infection.

OSHA and the CDC have set safety standards and precautions that protect employees in situations where they could be exposed to bloodborne pathogens. Precautions include proper hand washing, wearing gloves, and proper handling and disposing of sharp instruments and any other items that may have been contaminated by blood or other body fluids **(Figure 4–9)**. It is important that specific procedures be followed if blood or body fluid is present.

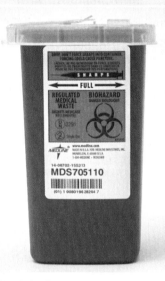

Fig. 4-9: Sharps containers are puncture-proof plastic biohazard containers for disposable needles and anything sharp and must be disposed of as medical waste.

Blood Exposure

You should never perform a service on a client with an open wound, rash, or abrasion. However, sometimes accidents happen while a service is being performed.

An **exposure incident** is contact with non-intact (broken) skin, blood, body fluid, or other potentially infectious materials that is the result of the performance of a worker's duties. Should the client suffer a cut or abrasion that bleeds during a service, follow the steps outlined in **Procedure 4-5: Handling an Exposure Incident: Client Injury** for the client's safety as well as your own.

Perform:

Perform 4-5: Handling an Exposure Incident: Client Injury

Note that some states require you to apply powdered alum, styptic powder, or a cyanoacrylate to an open wound with a disposable cotton-tipped instrument. In these cases, you should also immediately and securely discard the cotton-tipped instrument after application.[2]

As an eyelash technician, accidentally cutting yourself on the job is a real possibility. If you do suffer a cut and blood is present, you must follow the steps for an exposure incident outlined in **Procedure 4-6: Handling an Exposure Incident: Employee Injury**. Many of the steps are similar to those followed after a client injury, although attending to yourself should hopefully require fewer soft skills!

Perform:

Perform 4-6: Handling an Exposure Incident: Employee Injury

Personal Protective Equipment (PPE)

Many chemicals used in the salon or spa bear labels indicating that the use of PPE, such as gloves and safety glasses, is required when working with the products. Some equipment, such as gloves and masks, offer general protection from exposure to pathogens and should be worn whenever practical.

GLOVES

Gloves are single-use equipment; a new set is used for every client, and at times they must be changed during the service, according to protocol. Removal of gloves is performed by inverting the cuffs, pulling them off inside out, and disposing of them into the trash. The glove taken off first is held in the hand with a glove still on it; the glove with the cuff inverted is then pulled over the first glove inside out **(Figure 4–10)**. The first glove is then inside the second one, which has the service side now on the inside against the other glove, and they are disposed of together.

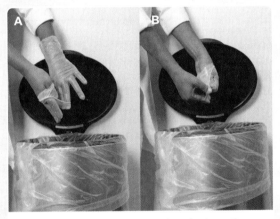

Fig. 4-10: First, remove one glove by inverting the cuff and pulling it off inside out (A). Then, with the cuff inverted, pull the second glove off over the inside-out first glove (B). Dispose of both gloves together.

If a service requires moving from one place of service to another several times or requires working on different body parts several sets of gloves will need to be used. The technician should wash their hands after removing each set of gloves and before putting on a new set when two services are being performed together, or use antimicrobial gel cleanser between sets of gloves during the same appointment.

 Caution!

When choosing which type of disposable gloves to use, you should avoid latex due to common allergies to the material. You should also exercise caution when using petroleum-based products, as petroleum-based gloves degrade on contact and cannot maintain a safe barrier. Nitrile gloves are the best alternative in both instances.

MASKS

Although you as an eyelash technician will not have much need of dust protection, properly fitted dust masks rated N95 are highly effective against germs and the respiratory droplets and aerosols that cause diseases such as COVID-19. However, N95 masks are *not* effective against chemical fumes or vapors.

Eyewash Stations

Ensure an eyewash station or kit is available in your treatment area or nearby and is accessible in your workplace. Be prepared to use the eyewash or eyewash kit if glue, tint, or lamination chemicals accidentally get into the client's eye; if watering of the eyes occurs due to glue fumes; or if there is any emergency where an immediate rinse is needed **(Figure 4–11)**. In cases where any amount of adhesive enters the eye, irrigate with an eyewash and then contact your client's eye doctor. Do not force the eyelids apart if they have become glued together.

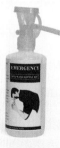

Fig. 4-11: In an emergency, use an eyewash station or kit and then contact a medical professional.

Check In

7. Why is it of the utmost importance to practice strict infection control protocols with every client?

....

....

Workbook Assessment

Fill in the Blank

Fill in the blanks below using words from the provided word bank.

QUESTION 18:

.... are the guidelines published by the Centers for Disease Control and Prevention (CDC) that insist that human blood and other body fluids must be considered potentially infectious.

QUESTION 19:

Aiofe goes to her regular eyelash technician for an eyelash service. When leaving the salon, Aiofe asks the technician if there is a place nearby where she can get takeout soup for her roommate who has the flu. A day later, the lash technician gets the symptoms of the flu. The technician concludes that though Aiofe seemed well, she must have been carrying the flu virus. In the given scenario, Aiofe is a(n)

.... carrier of the virus.

QUESTION 20:

The two organizations that have set the safety standards to be followed and precautions to be taken when there is a possibility of exposure to bloodborne pathogens are the Occupational Safety and Health Administration (OSHA) and the

................, or ....

QUESTION 21:

.... containers are plastic biohazard containers that are puncture-proof and are used for disposables, such as needles or razors.

QUESTION 22:

If, while performing their duties, a worker comes in contact with broken skin, blood or any other body fluids, or other infectious materials, the event is referred

to as a(n) ....

Word Bank

asymptomatic
exposure incident
CDC
eyewash
personal protective
N95
petroleum-based
Centers for Disease Control and Prevention
nitrile
sharps
fumes
latex
Standard Precautions

Ch. 04: Client Safety and Infection Control

QUESTION 23:

Many of the chemicals used in an eyelash salon require technicians to wear

.... equipment, such as masks, gloves, and safety glasses.

QUESTION 24:

Matías uses petroleum-based products in eyelash services. To ensure that the gloves do not get compromised because of degradation, Matías must not use

.... gloves. To minimize the chances of allergic reactions to the gloves,

Matías must also avoid using .... gloves. Matías can use .... gloves to avoid both the issues.

QUESTION 25:

Masks that are rated .... are very effective in protecting a person from respiratory droplets and germs, but they do not protect against chemical

.... and vapors.

QUESTION 26:

During an eyelash service, if you accidently flick a drop of lash glue in the client's eye,

you must immediately take the client to a(n) .... station and irrigate the eye with an eyewash before calling the eye doctor.

Ch. 04: Client Safety and Infection Control

Chapter Glossary

asymptomatic *A-simp-toe-**MA**-tick*	p. 064	showing no symptoms or signs of infection
exposure incident *ek-**SPOW**-zhur **IN**-sih-dent*	p. 064	contact with non-intact (broken) skin, blood, body fluid, or other potentially infectious materials that is the result of the performance of a worker's duties
Safety Data Sheet (SDS) ***SAYF**-tee **DAY**-tuh sheet*	p. 060	required by law for all products sold; SDSs include safety information about products compiled by the manufacturer, including hazardous ingredients, safe use and handling procedures, proper disposal guidelines, and precautions to reduce the risk of accidental harm or overexposure
sterilization *steh-rih-luh-**ZAY**-shun*	p. 057	process that destroys all microbial life, including spores; requires use of an autoclave or flash sterilizer

Procedure 4-1: Proper Hand Washing

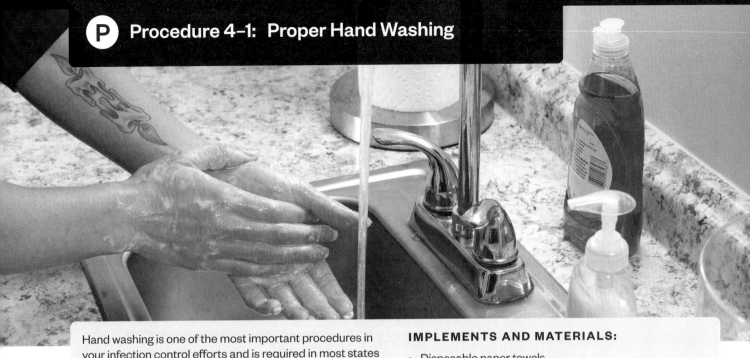

Hand washing is one of the most important procedures in your infection control efforts and is required in most states before beginning any service and after eating, smoking, or using the restroom.

IMPLEMENTS AND MATERIALS:

- Disposable paper towels
- Liquid soap in a pump container
- Nail brush

PROCEDURE:

STEP 1
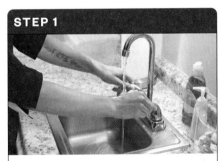
Turn the water on and wet your hands.

STEP 2
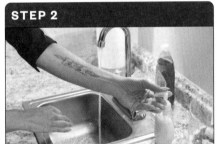
Pump soap from a pump container onto the palm of your hand.

STEP 3
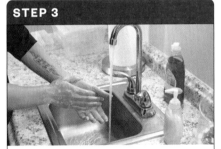
Rub your hands together, all over and vigorously, until a lather forms. Continue for a minimum of 20 seconds.

STEP 4
Scrub your nails with a nail brush if product or debris is visible under your nails or if you are washing your hands following an exposure incident.

STEP 4A
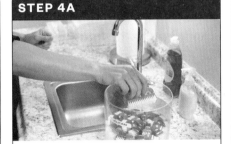
Choose a clean and disinfected nail brush.

STEP 4B
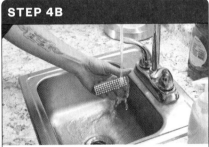
Wet the nail brush and pump soap onto the bristles.

Ch. 04: Client Safety and Infection Control

Procedure 4-1: Proper Hand Washing

STEP 4C
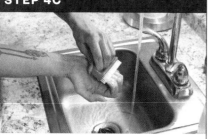
Brush your nails horizontally back and forth under the free edges.

STEP 4D
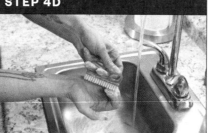
Change the direction of the brush to vertical and move the brush up and down along the nail folds of the fingernails. The process for brushing both hands should take about 60 seconds to complete.

STEP 4E
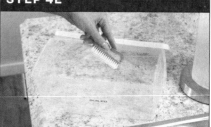
Rinse the nail brush and deposit it in a labeled container for dirty implements.

STEP 5
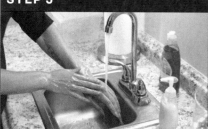
Rinse your hands in warm running water.

STEP 6
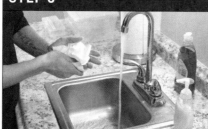
Use a clean cloth or paper towel to dry your hands, according to the salon or spa's policies or state rules and regulations.

STEP 7
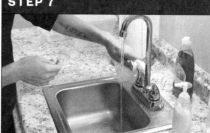
After drying your hands, turn off the water with the towel. Use the towel to open the door and then dispose of the towel. Touching a doorknob with your bare fingers can recontaminate your hands.

Procedure 4–2: Cleaning and Disinfecting Nonporous, Reusable Items

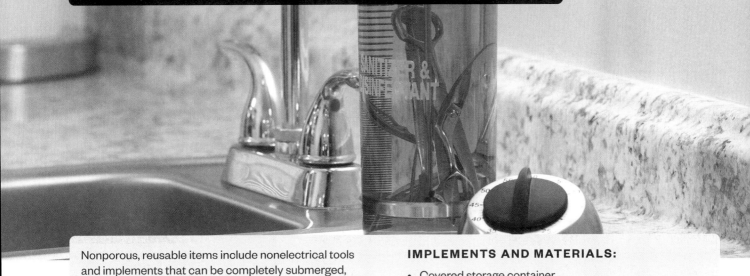

Nonporous, reusable items include nonelectrical tools and implements that can be completely submerged, such as tweezers and trimming scissors, as well as larger equipment that cannot be submerged, all the way up to nonporous work surfaces.

IMPLEMENTS AND MATERIALS:

- Covered storage container
- Disinfectant solution, spray, or wipes
- Disposable gloves
- Disposable towels
- Liquid soap or cleaning solution
- Safety glasses
- Scrub brush
- Timer
- Tongs

PROCEDURE:

STEP 1

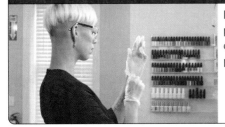

It is important to wear safety glasses and gloves while cleaning and disinfecting to protect your eyes from unintentional splashes of disinfectant, to prevent possible contamination of the implements by your hands, and to protect your hands from the powerful chemicals in the disinfectant solution.

STEP 2

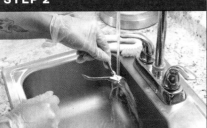

Rinse items with warm running water.

STEP 3

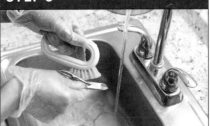

Use a small scrubbing brush to wash items with soap or cleaning solution.

STEP 4

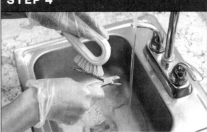

Brush grooved items thoroughly and open hinged implements to scrub the revealed areas clean.

Ch. 04: Client Safety and Infection Control

Procedure 4-2: Cleaning and Disinfecting Nonporous, Reusable Items

STEP 5

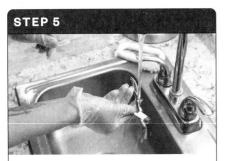

Rinse away all traces of soap or solution with clean running water. Soap is most easily rinsed off in warm, not hot, water.

STEP 6

Dry items with a clean or disposable towel.

STEP 7

Disinfect items as appropriate or required by your state.

STEP 7A

Immersion is used for items that can be safely and effectively immersed in disinfectant.

STEP 7A (1)

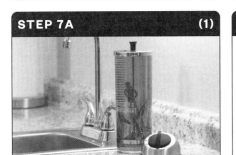

Completely immerse cleaned items in an appropriate disinfection container holding an EPA-registered disinfectant approved for use in your state for the required time listed in the manufacturer's instructions. Remember to open hinged implements before immersing them in the disinfectant. If the disinfectant solution is visibly dirty, or if the solution has been contaminated, it must be replaced.

STEP 7A (2)

After the required contact time has passed, remove items from the disinfectant solution with tongs or gloved hands, rinse in warm running water, and dry thoroughly with a disposable towel or allow to air dry on a clean towel. Do not store implements with any moisture on them, particularly in the hinges.

STEP 7B

Sprays are used for larger tools and implements that cannot or should not be immersed.

STEP 7B (1)

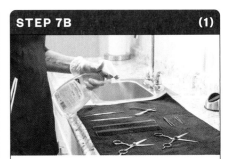

Place cleaned items on a disinfected surface or clean towel and spray with disinfectant until thoroughly saturated. Ensure that all surfaces of items stay visibly moist for the full contact time listed on the label.

STEP 7B (2)

After the required contact time has passed, pick up items with tongs or gloved hands, rinse in warm running water, and pat dry.

STEP 7C

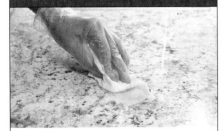

Wipes are used for surfaces and other nonsubmersible items.

  i. Steps 2 through 6 are not required when using one wipe to clean and a second wipe to disinfect.
  ii. Use an EPA-registered wipe to wipe surfaces or items and ensure that all surfaces remain visibly moist for the contact time listed on the label.

STEP 8

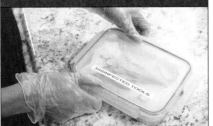

Store items as directed by your state rules. Most states require that dry, disinfected items be stored in a clean, covered container labeled "disinfected" or "ready to use" until needed.

STEP 9

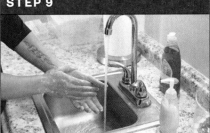

Remove gloves and thoroughly wash your hands with warm running water and liquid soap. Rinse and dry hands with a clean fabric or disposable towel.

Procedure 4-3: Pre-Service Procedure

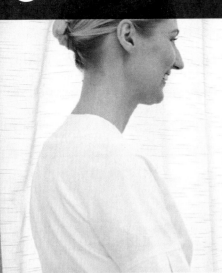
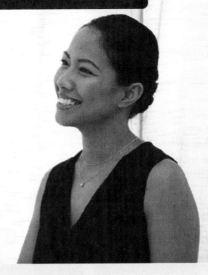

IMPLEMENTS AND MATERIALS:

Actual equipment, materials, and products will vary depending on the client's service.

EQUIPMENT:

- Autoclave
- Client charts
- Close-lid garbage cans
- Covered containers for applicators, mascara wands, cotton pads
- Covered holding tray for disinfectant solution
- Adjustable LED light
- Technician's chair
- Treatment table
- Trolley or rolling cart

SUPPLIES:

- Bed sheets, 2 twin-size flat
- Bolster
- Dental mirror
- Dish soap
- Distilled water
- EPA-registered disinfectant
- Emergency eyewash kit
- Facial cape for draping
- Fine felt-tipped marker
- Hand sanitizer and liquid soap
- Hand towels (2 to 4)
- Hand-held mirror
- Jade stones or adhesive holder
- Lash tile or palette
- Linens
- Eyelash separation tool
- Mini fan, bulb syringe, or nano mister
- Pillows
- Plastic mixing cup
- Small bowl
- Squeeze bottle with distilled water
- Timer
- Trimming scissors
- Tweezers (straight pointed, curved, boot tip, slanted tip)

SINGLE-USE ITEMS:

- Adhesive stickers for jade stones and lash tiles
- Assortment of individual eyelash extensions
- Assortment of artificial temporary individual eyelashes
- Assortment of artificial temporary strip eyelashes
- Assortment of artificial temporary cluster eyelashes
- Assortment of silicone lash lift shields or rods
- Cotton rounds or squares (pads)
- Cotton swabs
- Esthetics wipes (4" × 4" for cleansing)
- Eyelash cleansing brushes
- Eyebrow lamination kit (brow bonder, neutralizing solution, product tray, post-treatment lotion)
- Eyelash lift kit (includes lash y-comb, lash lift adhesive, lash lift solution, neutralizing solution, product tray, post-treatment lotion)
- Eyelash or eyebrow tint kit (assorted colors of black and brown)
- Gloves
- Glue rings and glue cups
- Hair clips
- Headband or protective cap
- Interdental brushes
- Lint-free applicators
- Mascara brushes
- Micro swabs
- Plastic cling wrap
- Paper drapes
- Paper towels
- Protective paper

Ch. 04: Client Safety and Infection Control

Procedure 4-3: Pre-Service Procedure

- Surgical paper tape (regular and sensitive)
- Trash bag
- Treatment table paper rolls
- Under-eye gel pads
- Petroleum jelly/occlusive cream
- Temporary eyelash adhesive

PRODUCTS:

- Eyelash cleanser
- Eyelash adhesive remover
- Eyelash extension adhesive
- Eyelash primer (optional)
- Longer life coating sealant (optional for classic extensions)

In the morning, the treatment room should be ready from the previous night's thorough cleaning and disinfecting. Perform the preparations listed below between every client service.

PROCEDURE:

A. Preparing the Treatment Room

STEP 1

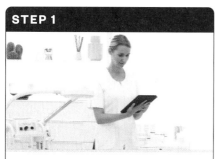

Review your client schedule to refresh your mind about each repeat client you see that day and their concerns. Ensure you have enough of all the products you will use for the remainder of the day.

STEP 2

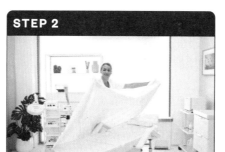

Check your room supply of linens (towels and sheets) and replenish as needed. Change the treatment chair or table linens.

STEP 3

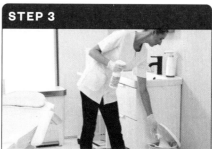

Throw away disposables used during the previous service.

STEP 4

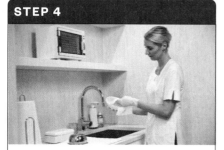

Clean and disinfect used implements, such as tweezers, dental mirror, jade stone, lash tile, and trimming scissors.

STEP 5

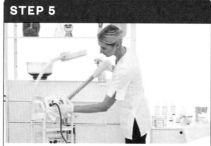

Clean and disinfect machine parts used during the previous service, counters, and the adjustable lamp.

STEP 6

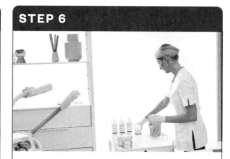

Refill needed disposable supplies, such as gloves, eyelash extensions, lifting kits, lamination kits, tint kits, under-eye gel pads, surgical paper tape, mascara brushes, micro swabs, interdental brushes, lint-free applicators, cotton pads, and cotton swabs.

Procedure 4-3: Pre-Service Procedure

B. Preparing for the Client

STEP 7
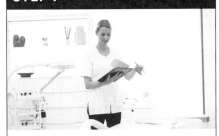
Retrieve and review the client's intake form and service record card. If the client is new, let the receptionist know they will need an intake form.

STEP 8
Take care of your personal needs and appearance before the client arrives—use the restroom, drink water, return a personal call, check yourself in a mirror. When your client arrives, place your full attention on their needs. Double-check your room, including cleanliness, music, and temperature.

STEP 9
Silence your cell phone. Eliminate anything that can distract you from your client.

STEP 10
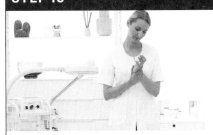
Take a few deep breaths, stretch, clear your head of personal concerns and issues, and remember you are committed to providing your clients with fantastic services and your full attention.

STEP 11
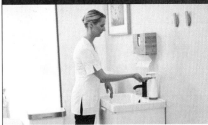
Wash your hands before greeting your client. Reference **Procedure 4–1: Proper Hand Washing.**

STEP 12
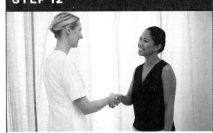
Greet your client in the reception area with a warm smile and handshake in a professional manner. Introduce yourself if you've never met. Ask them for the completed intake form.

STEP 13
If the client is new, ask any questions you have concerning the intake form. If the client is returning, ask them if anything has changed since their last visit, such as new medications or medical diagnoses, other eyelash or eyebrow treatments not done by you, or the use of new products. Ask how their eyelashes or eyebrows have been since the last treatment.

STEP 14
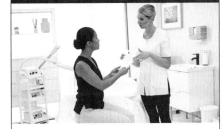
Indicate where to securely place personal items. Changing clothes is unnecessary—clothing can be protected with proper towel draping. Ask the client to remove all jewelry that would inhibit the service and put it in a safe place.

STEP 15
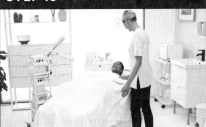
Invite the client to take a seat in the treatment chair or lie down on the treatment table.

Procedure 4-3: Pre-Service Procedure

STEP 16

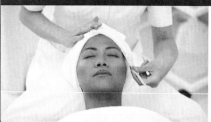

Drape the client properly and place the hair in a protective cap or use a headband and towels to drape the hair. Ensure their comfort before beginning the service.

STEP 17

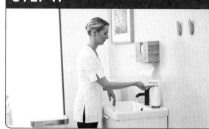

Again, briefly explain the treatment plan to the client and ask/answer any remaining questions. Wash your hands with soap and warm water as detailed in **Procedure 4-1: Proper Hand Washing**. Always wash your hands and put on gloves before starting any treatment.

STEP 18

Proceed with the next steps in your service.

Procedure 4-4: Post-Service Procedure

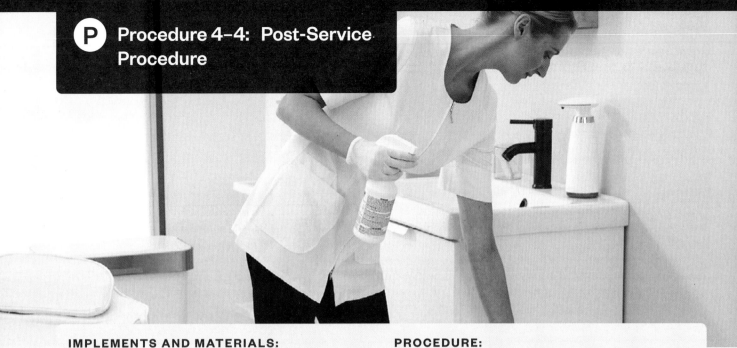

IMPLEMENTS AND MATERIALS:

Refer to the items listed for **Procedure 4-3: Pre-Service Procedure.**
At the end of the service, you must clean the treatment room and prepare it for your next client.

PROCEDURE:

A. Advise the Client and Promote Products

STEP 1

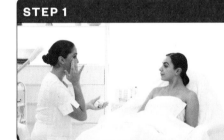

After the treatment, ask how the client feels as well as how the eyelashes or eyebrows feel. Ask if they have any questions or concerns. Determine a plan for future visits.

STEP 2

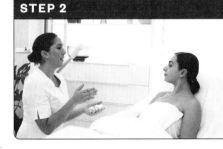

Outline proper home care and how the recommended professional products will help with eyelash extension retention. Explain each home care product step by step.

Ch. 04: Client Safety and Infection Control

Procedure 4-4: Post-Service Procedure

B. Schedule the Next Appointment and Thank the Client

STEP 3

Escort the client to the reception desk. Write a service ticket for today's service, recommended products, and when the next service should be. Place all recommended home care products on the counter.

STEP 4

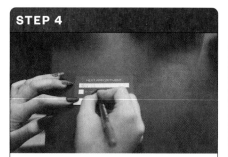

After the client has paid for their service and take-home products, ask if you can schedule the next appointment. Write the next appointment time on your business card. Set up a reminder call, text message, or e-mail according to your client's preference at least 24 to 48 hours in advance of the next appointment.

STEP 5

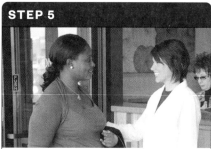

Thank the client for the opportunity to work together. Encourage the client to contact you with any questions. Thank the client again, shake hands, and give a friendly send-off.

STEP 6

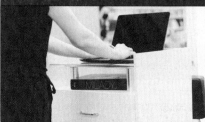

Record service information, observations, and product recommendations on the service record card. If your salon uses a paper system, return the service record card for filing with the completed client intake form.

C. At the End of the Service

STEP 7

Put on a fresh pair of gloves.

STEP 8

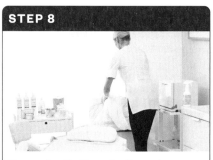

Place all soiled laundry linens in a covered receptacle.

STEP 9

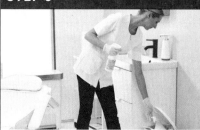

Discard any used disposables into a covered trash container.

STEP 10

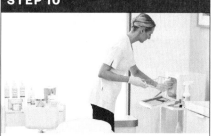

Clean trolley and workstation surfaces.

Procedure 4-4: Post-Service Procedure

STEP 11

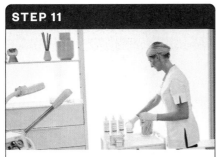

Reset products and disposable items and replenish clean headbands and towel wraps.

STEP 12

Use an antibacterial dish soap and warm water to wash any used bowls. Rinse and dry thoroughly.

STEP 13

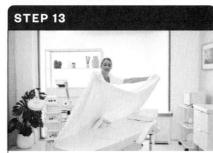

Change the linen on the treatment table.

D. At the End of the Day

STEP 14

Put on a fresh pair of gloves. Turn off and unplug all equipment.

STEP 15

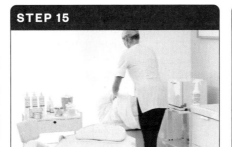

Remove all dirty laundry from the hamper. Spray the hamper with a disinfectant spray or wipe it down with disinfectant to prevent mildew growth.

STEP 16

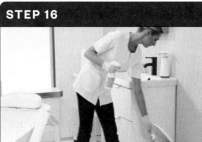

Discard all used single-use brushes, utensils, and supplies. Empty the waste container and place a clean liner inside.

STEP 17

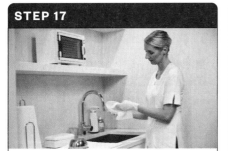

Thoroughly clean and disinfect all multiuse tools and implements.

STEP 18

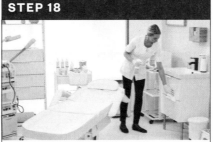

Clean and disinfect all counters, the treatment chair, machines, other furniture, and the adjustable LED lamp.

STEP 19

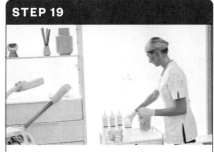

Replenish the room with fresh linens, tools, utensils, and other supplies for the next day.

STEP 20

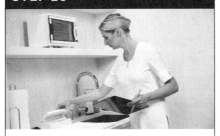

Change the disinfectant solution.

STEP 21

Check the room for dirt, smudges, or dust on the walls, on the baseboards, on the air vents, and in corners. Vacuum and mop the room with a disinfectant. Optional: Spray the air in the room with a disinfectant aerosol spray.

Procedure 4–5: Handling an Exposure Incident: Client Injury

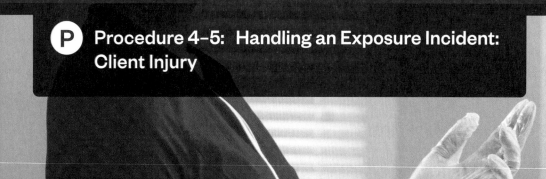

Should you accidentally cut a client during a service, calmly take the following steps. These guidelines apply to all services in the beauty and wellness industry.

IMPLEMENTS AND MATERIALS:

- Antiseptic
- Bandages
- Disposable gloves
- Disposable paper towels
- Liquid soap
- Plastic bag
- Disinfectant solution, spray, or wipes
- Sharps box (optional)

PROCEDURE:

STEP 1
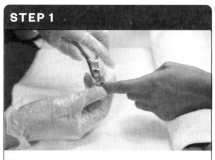
Stop the service immediately.

STEP 2
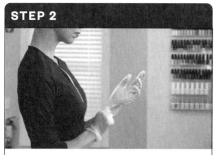
Put on gloves (if you were not already wearing gloves for the procedure).

STEP 3
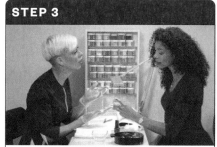
Face your client and calmly apologize for the incident.

STEP 4
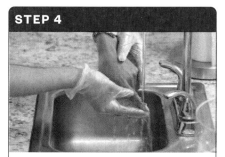
If appropriate, assist your client to the sink, wash the injured area with soap, and rinse it under running water.

STEP 5
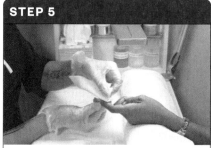
Pat the injured area dry using a new, clean paper towel.

STEP 6
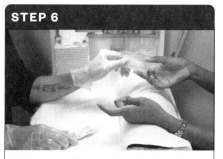
Offer your client antiseptic and an adhesive bandage.

Procedure 4-5: Handling an Exposure Incident: Client Injury

STEP 7

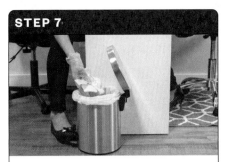

Discard all single-use contaminated objects, such as wipes or cotton balls, in a plastic bag and then place in a trash bag. Deposit sharp disposables in a sharps box. Dispose of double-bagged items and sharps containers as required by state or local law. In general, all these items (except sharps) may go into the regular trash.

STEP 8

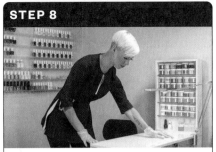

Remove all implements from the workstation and then clean and disinfect workstation surfaces.

STEP 9

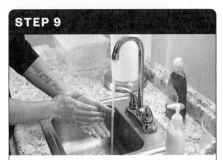

Discard gloves and thoroughly wash hands with warm running water and liquid soap. Rinse and dry hands with a clean fabric or disposable towel and then put on fresh gloves.

STEP 10

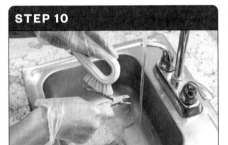

Properly clean and disinfect implements.

STEP 11

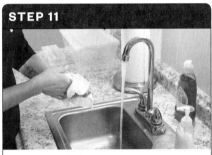

Discard gloves and thoroughly wash your hands with warm running water and liquid soap. Rinse and dry hands with a clean fabric or disposable towel and return to the service.

STEP 12

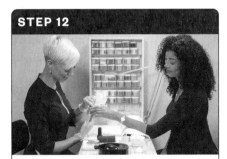

Recommend that the client see a physician if any signs of redness, swelling, pain, or irritation develop. Ask if the client would like to continue the service and return to where you left off if they are willing. If you were working on the client's hands and they have refused a bandage, put on gloves before finishing the service.

Ch. 04: Client Safety and Infection Control

Procedure 4–6: Handling an Exposure Incident: Employee Injury

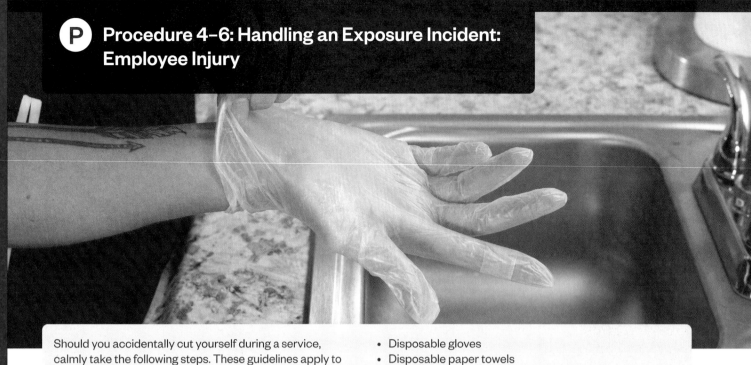

Should you accidentally cut yourself during a service, calmly take the following steps. These guidelines apply to all services in the beauty and wellness industry.

IMPLEMENTS AND MATERIALS:

- Antiseptic
- Bandages
- Cotton
- Disposable gloves
- Disposable paper towels
- Liquid soap
- Plastic bag
- Disinfectant solution, spray, or wipes
- Sharps box (optional)

PROCEDURE:

STEP 1

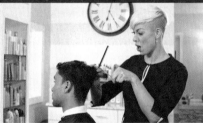

Stop the service immediately.

STEP 2

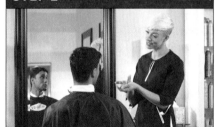

Inform your client of what has happened. Let them know you are taking care of your cut and that the service will be interrupted for a few minutes. If the nature of your cut is severe, ask an employee to assist with the exposure incident.

STEP 3

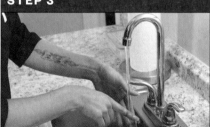

If appropriate, wash and rinse the injured area under running water.

Procedure 4-6: Handling an Exposure Incident: Employee Injury

STEP 4

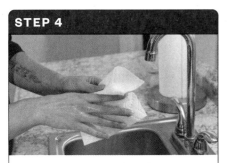

Pat the injured area dry using a new, clean paper towel.

STEP 5

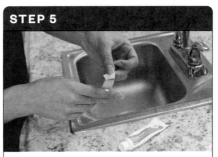

Apply antiseptic and an adhesive bandage to the wound.

STEP 6

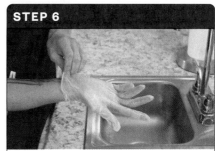

Put on gloves.

STEP 7

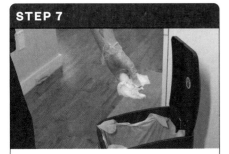

Discard all single-use contaminated objects, such as wipes or cotton balls, in a plastic bag and then place in a trash bag. Deposit sharp disposables in a sharps box. Dispose of double-bagged items and sharps containers as required by state or local law. In general, all these items (except sharps) may go into the regular trash.

STEP 8

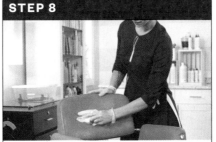

Remove all implements from the workstation and then clean and disinfect workstation surfaces.

STEP 9

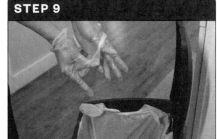

Discard gloves and thoroughly wash hands with warm running water and liquid soap. Rinse and dry hands with a clean fabric or disposable towel and then put on fresh gloves.

STEP 10

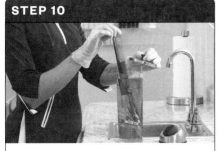

Properly clean and disinfect implements.

STEP 11

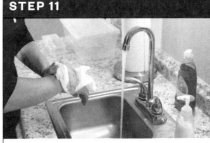

Discard gloves and thoroughly wash your hands with warm running water and liquid soap. Rinse and dry hands with a clean fabric or disposable towel.

STEP 12

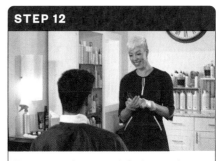

Return to where you left the service.

Ch. 04: Client Safety and Infection Control

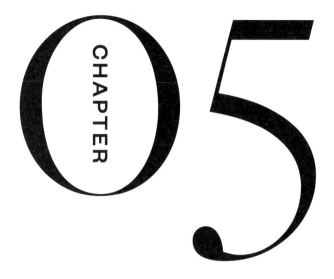

CHAPTER 05

Tools, Products, and Ingredients

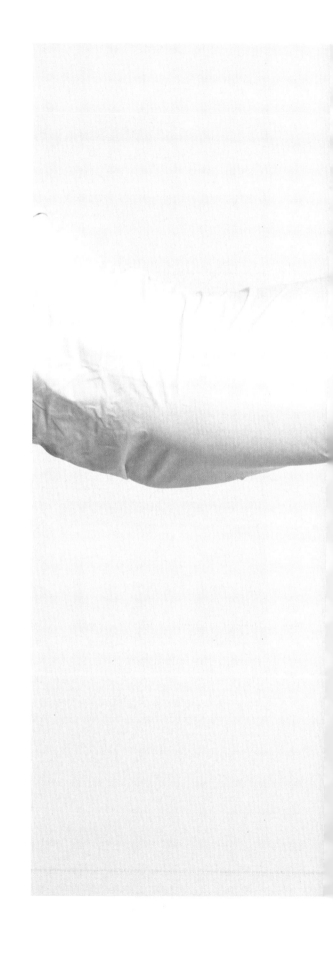

🚩 Learning Objectives

After completing this chapter, you will be able to:

1. Explain why knowledge of eyelash extension tools, products, and ingredients is essential to eyelash extension technicians.
2. Describe eyelash adhesive ingredients and how to properly use and store them.
3. Identify the implements, tools, and equipment required for eyelash and eyebrow services.
4. Compare the different eyelash extension options.
5. Recognize the professional products used during an eyelash or eyebrow service.

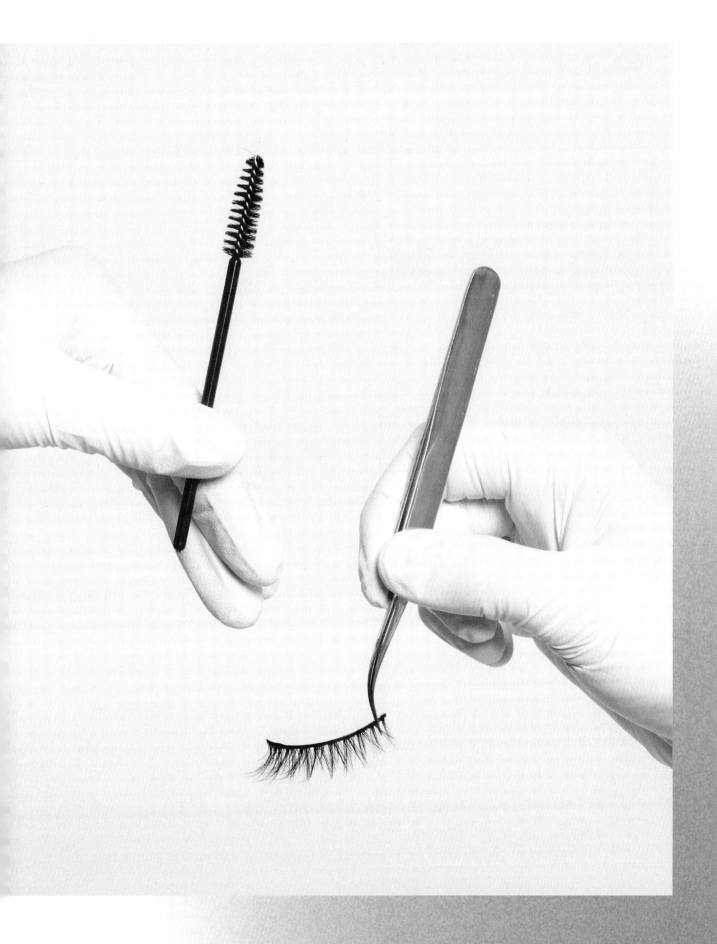

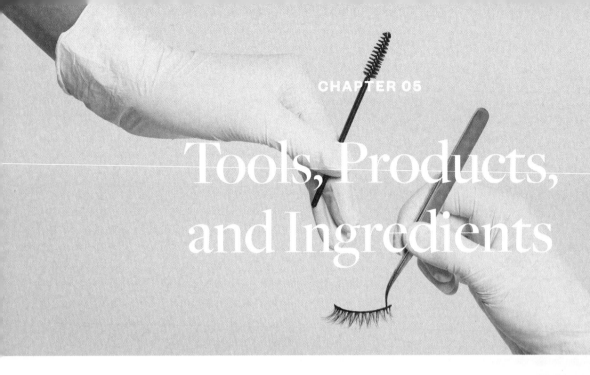

CHAPTER 05

Tools, Products, and Ingredients

Why Study Tools, Products, and Ingredients?

 Learning Objective 01

Explain why knowledge of eyelash extension tools, products, and ingredients is essential to eyelash extension technicians.

Using the proper tools and ingredients when performing eyelash and eyebrow services is key to providing long-lasting extensions and effective chemical services for your client. You will need to learn the different types of adhesives, single- and multiuse tools and implements, eyelash extension options, and chemical service ingredients. This knowledge will help you make the best choices when it comes to application, infection control, consultation, and lash retention. In other words, all key areas of eyelash and eyebrow services.

Eyelash technicians should study and have a thorough understanding of eyelash extension tools, products, and ingredients because:

- Eyelash extension adhesives are affected by both humidity and temperature in ways that directly impact lash retention.
- Some tools and implements used in eyelash and eyebrow services can be disinfected and reused, whereas others cannot be.
- There are many different extension types and options to choose among to meet client needs and budgets.
- Using service products correctly and safely comes from recognizing their ingredients and the effect they have on the lashes and skin around them.

 Check In

1. Why do you think it is important to study eyelash extension tools, products, and ingredients?

Adhesives

Learning Objective 02

Describe eyelash adhesive ingredients and how to properly use and store them.

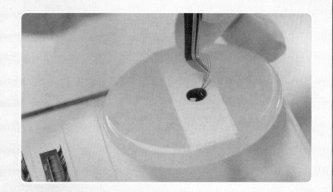

Eyelash adhesive is used to make artificial eyelashes stick to the natural lash line or the natural lash, depending on which type of artificial lashes are being applied. Understanding how adhesives work ensures not only lash retention but also client safety.

Eyelash Extension Adhesive

Eyelash extensions are applied to the natural lash using eyelash extension adhesive. The typical shelf life of adhesive is four to five weeks. Once it is open, it is good until it starts looking stringy or cloudy. A good practice to make sure your glue lasts is to clean the bottle tip with a lint-free wipe and securely fasten the adhesive cover when you're done using it. Always be sure to check the manufacturer's recommendations, as different brands suggest different storage areas based on temperature.

Here's a Tip

It is important to shake eyelash adhesive before dispensing so that you properly mix all the ingredients!

INGREDIENTS

Eyelash extension adhesive is mainly comprised of cyanoacrylate, along with stabilizing agents, coloring agents, thickeners, and other compounds, such as latex.

- **Cyanoacrylate**, the main component of eyelash extension adhesives, is an acrylate monomer that is cured and used as an adhesive. Although there are several types of cyanoacrylates, only some are used for eyelash extension adhesives. They vary by their adhesion qualities and by the level of fumes they give off while curing.

Methyl-Cyanoacrylate	Considered industrial grade and should never be used for eyelash extension adhesive, as it can cause permanent blindness.
Ethyl-Cyanoacrylate	Considered medical grade and is used the most for eyelash extension adhesive because of its strong adhesion.
Butyl-Cyanoacrylate	Considered medical grade and is used for sensitive eyelash extension adhesives. Although it has a longer drying time and the adhesion is not as strong as ethyl-cyanoacrylate, it is considered low odor.
Methoxy-Cyanoacrylate	Considered medical grade but should not be used for eyelash extension adhesive because, although it has the least odor, the adhesive quality is too low for good lash retention.

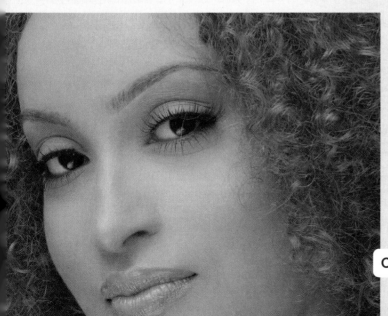

> **Caution!**
>
> Be prepared to use the emergency eye flush station should adhesive contact the eye. The eye flush procedure consists of holding the lids of the affected eye open and placing the eye, head down and turned to the side, under gently running water from a faucet, eye wash station, or eye wash kit for approximately five minutes. If irritation does not resolve, recommend or seek medical attention.

- **Formaldehyde**, a colorless gas with a strong odor, is a byproduct of curing cyanoacrylates. Fumes will be given off by any lash adhesive containing cyanoacrylates, even if in just trace amounts.[1]
- **Polymethyl methacrylate (PMMA)**, used as a thickening agent, is a synthetic resin produced from the polymerization of methyl methacrylate. It assists in the adhesion of the extension to the natural lash.[2]
- **Hydroquinone**, used as a stabilizing agent, keeps the cyanoacrylate from curing in the bottle by stopping the polymerization process.[3] Although it makes up a very small percentage of adhesives, hydroquinone can cause skin irritation and skin discoloration.[4]
- **Carbon black**, a dark black powder used as a pigment, is used as a coloring agent. The Food and Drug Administration (FDA) has found that this ingredient should *not* be used in the eye area; however, it is still used in many cosmetics, such as mascaras and eyeliners.[5] Carbon black has been linked to increased incidence of cancer and negative effects on body organs.[6] There are clear eyelash adhesives that do not contain carbon black, as an alternative for clients with sensitivities or those who do not wish to be exposed to it.

> **Caution!**
>
> Cyanoacrylate allergic reactions can be difficult to distinguish from general irritation and can occur even if the skin doesn't come in contact with adhesive.

DRYING VERSUS CURING

To ensure proper application, the adhesive must be completely dried *and* cured. Drying occurs quickly when the ingredients toward the outside of the lash adhesive evaporate into the air. As the adhesive hardens, this allows the technician to continue lashing without lashes clumping or sticking together. To allow for maximum dry time between lashes, it's recommended to work on the eyes alternatively and to apply extensions to different parts of the lash line. A mini fan is a great way to assist in drying time.

Curing occurs when the adhesive completely dries in the center by taking in the moisture in the air. Through the chemical process of **polymerization**, the cyanoacrylate monomers form bonds with water, which acts as the *catalyst*, to create long molecular chains. This turns the liquid adhesive into a solid that binds the eyelash extension with the natural lash. Curing takes longer than drying, typically a full day to do so. Lash technicians should remind clients to not allow their lashes to get wet until the curing process is completed. Tools to assist the curing process are nano misters and nebulizers, which are used to mist applied extensions **(Figure 5–1)**.

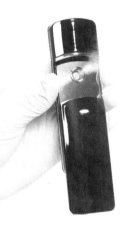

Fig. 5-1: A nano mister.

HUMIDITY AND TEMPERATURE

Humidity and temperature are important factors in the dry time of lash extensions and can affect retention. Humidity, the amount of moisture present in the air, affects how quickly the cyanoacrylate in the adhesive cures, whereas temperature affects the viscosity, and therefore drying time, of the adhesive.

High Humidity	Cyanoacrylate in adhesive cures too quickly from the high amount of moisture in the air. Can cause the adhesive drop used during the service to dry before application, creating a weak bond between the natural lash and the extension and resulting in poor retention.
Low Humidity	Cyanoacrylate in adhesive cures too slowly, or not at all, from not being able to draw enough moisture from the surrounding air. Can cause applied extensions to stick to other lashes and clump, which in turn can cause damage to the client's natural lashes as well as create an increased chance of sensitivity from the fumes. A quick fix to low humidity when applying extensions is to use a nano mister or nebulizer to cure the adhesive.
High Temperature	Adhesive becomes too thin and drying time lessens. Can cause issues with an adhesive drop for application to dry too quickly and result in poor retention.
Lower Temperature	Adhesive becomes too thick and drying time lengthens. Can cause issues with applied extensions sticking to other lashes and clumping.

Ensure an ideal humidity level in your salon by investing in:

- a hygrometer, a tool to measure humidity;
- a dehumidifier, a device to reduce and maintain humidity levels; and
- a humidifier, a device to increase and maintain humidity levels.

Here's a Tip

The ideal humidity levels of the area you are working in should be between 40 and 60 percent, and the temperature should stay at a moderate 70 degrees Fahrenheit (21 degrees Celsius).

Clients should avoid hot and humid temperatures outside and inside buildings within 24 hours of having eyelash extensions applied. Examples are cooking over a stove or taking a hot bath. Good advice for clients who cannot avoid high-humidity environments may be to carry a small fan or keep their vehicle and house at a cooler temperature.

STORAGE

Adhesives should be stored upright and in a dark, cool place. Manufacturers may recommend putting your lash adhesive in a refrigerator before opening, but once opened it is not recommended to store adhesive in a fridge as it causes the chemicals in the glue to clump inside the bottle. A bottle of adhesive should be replaced after four to five weeks, but always follow the manufacturer's suggested shelf life. If the adhesive is starting to look cloudy or stringy, it is best to toss it out and open a new bottle.

Here's a Tip

Always check the manufacturer's storage requirements for chemical products, including adhesives.

Ch. 05: Tools, Products, and Ingredients

Temporary Eyelash Adhesive

Temporary eyelashes, such as strip or cluster lashes, require a latex-based adhesive to adhere to the natural lash line **(Figure 5–2)**. Some clients may be allergic to the latex in this type of glue.

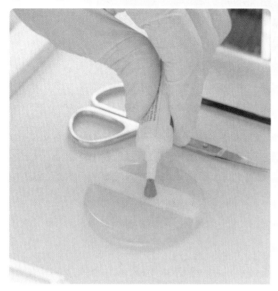

Fig. 5-2: Temporary eyelash adhesive.

When in doubt, give the client an allergy patch test by putting a drop of the adhesive behind one ear or in the crook of an elbow or behind the knee. Alternatively, attach a single individual eyelash to the base of the eyelash, being sure to not attach it to the skin. If there is no reaction within 24 hours, proceed with the application. Latex-free adhesives are available if needed.

> **⚠ Caution!**
>
> Never apply temporary strips, clusters, or individual lashes with eyelash extension adhesive. Temporary lashes are meant to be removed after hours of wear, not weeks.

✓ Check In

2. How long does it take for adhesive to cure?

3. How often should you change out your adhesive drop?

4. What effect does high humidity have on adhesives?

Workbook Assessment

Matching

For the following questions, match each statement to the correct letter choice.

QUESTION 1:

Match the different types of cyanoacrylates with their descriptions.

…………..) It is an industrial-grade adhesive that can cause permanent blindness.

…………..) It is a medical-grade adhesive that provides strong adhesion and is most commonly used in eyelash extension adhesives.

…………..) It is a medical-grade adhesive that does not provide very strong adhesion and is used for sensitive eyelash extension adhesives.

…………..) It is a medical-grade adhesive that is not suitable for eyelash extension adhesives as it provides very poor adhesion.

Choices

A. ethyl-cyanoacrylate
B. butyl-cyanoacrylate
C. methoxy-cyanoacrylate
D. methyl-cyanoacrylate

QUESTION 2:

Match the ingredients of eyelash extension adhesives with their roles.

…………..) the primary component of eyelash extension adhesives that provides adhesion

…………..) a pigment that is used as a coloring agent

…………..) a synthetic resin that acts as a thickening agent

…………..) a stabilizing agent that prevents the adhesive from curing in the bottle

Choices

A. carbon black
B. polymethyl methacrylate
C. hydroquinone
D. cyanoacrylate

Implements, Tools, and Equipment

 Learning Objective 03

Identify the implements, tools, and equipment required for eyelash and eyebrow services.

Implements are tools used to perform eyelash extension services, as well as eyelash and eyebrow chemical services. There are two types of implements used by technicians: multiuse, which can be properly cleaned and disinfected and reused for the life of the tool; and single use, which are disposable and discarded after one use.

Multiuse Tools

Multiuse implements, also known as *reusable implements*, must be properly cleansed and disinfected after each use. They are often made of metal. You should ideally have several clean and disinfected copies of a tool available at all times.

TWEEZERS

Tweezers are designed to assist in every step of your lash service, from isolating natural lashes to creating volume lash fans. The two most common materials used to make tweezers are stainless steel and titanium. Stainless steel tweezers are more resistant to rust, although rust can still happen if the tweezers are not properly cared for. Steel tweezers contain a small amount of nickel as well. It's rare, but nickel can cause an adverse reaction in some people. Titanium tweezers, on the other hand, are much lighter in weight and are totally rust-free. They are allergy free and commonly used in the medical field.

 Caution!

It is possible that a reaction can occur from stainless steel tweezers. Avoid directly contacting the client's skin with your tweezers.

There are many different types of tweezers based on their tips and purpose.

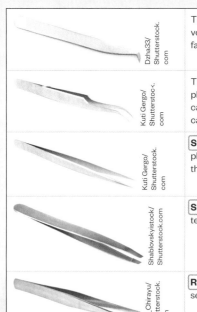

	Dzha33/Shutterstock.com	The **boot tip tweezer**, or *L-shaped tweezer*, has a sharply angled curved tip and is mainly used for volume and mega volume lashing. Due to its angled tip, it works well when creating and picking up lash fans.
	Kuti Gergo/Shutterstock.com	The **curved tweezer** has a gentle curved tip and is typically used for isolation as well as precision placement of lash extensions. The curve can allow for easier isolation closer to the client's eyelid. Be very careful when using curved tweezers when isolating natural lashes since the tips are pointed down and can poke the eye area!
	Kuti Gergo/Shutterstock.com	**Straight tweezers** are long and narrow, ending in a tapered point and are ideal for picking up and placing lash extensions. They can also be used for isolation. There are several types that fall within this category.
	Shablovskyistock/Shutterstock.com	**Slant tweezers** are typically used for eyebrow shaping; however, they can also be used for applying temporary strip or cluster eyelashes. The tip is blunt but has a slight slant ideal for gripping and holding.
	Chi_Chirayu/Shutterstock.com	**Round tweezers** have rounded tips that make it ideal for safely removing tape and eye pads after a service is completed.

Ch. 05: Tools, Products, and Ingredients

Typically, the tweezers you isolate with go into your non-dominant hand, and the tweezers you pick up and place eyelash extensions with go into your dominant hand. This is just a guide, and you should practice both ways to see what is more comfortable and accurate for you. To keep your tweezers in their best condition, keep them stored in a case when not in use. Remember that the tip is very fine and fragile and can become bent if dropped. If this happens, the tweezers will need to be replaced.

Here's a Tip

To prolong the life of your tweezers, remove any adhesive from the tweezers immediately. Check your tweezers often for damage. The quality of tweezers will also affect the amount of time it takes to complete an eyelash extension service.

EYELASH SEPARATION TOOL

The eyelash separation tool is used during an eyelash lifting (perming) service and is usually made of stainless steel **(Figure 5-3)**. The tip is a sharply angled pick. It is used to straighten and separate lashes after they have been adhered to the lash lift shields or rods.

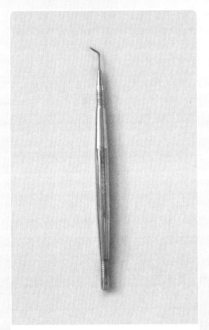

Fig. 5-3: Eyelash separation tool.

TRIMMING SCISSORS

Trimming scissors are used to trim eye pads if needed, are used to cut medical tape to place over lower lashes, and can be used to open product packaging easily.

Caution!

Never cut eye pads after you have placed them on the client!

LASH TILE OR LASH PALETTE

The lash tile or lash palette can be made of glass, crystal, or acrylic and is used to organize strips of lash extension **(Figure 5-4)**. Some palettes have lines and lash extension sizes etched into them already, whereas others you can write on yourself. Another feature of some tiles are small wells to be used for adhesive.

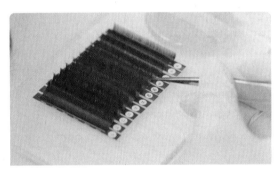

Fig. 5-4: Lash tile.

JADE STONE OR CRYSTAL

A jade stone or crystal serves as a tool to hold adhesives. It keeps the adhesive cool and prevents it from drying out too quickly. It can also be used to hold eyelash primers or adhesive removers. For infection control purposes and easy cleanup, layer two strips of medical tape or use a jade stone sticker on top of jade stone or crystal before applying adhesive.

Caution!

Check with your instructor or state board to see if jade stones are allowed in your state. Some states have banned the use of jade stones as they are made of a porous natural stone.

Ch. 05: Tools, Products, and Ingredients

MINI FAN, BULB SYRINGE, NANO MISTER, OR NEBULIZER

A mini fan or bulb syringe can be used to quicken the drying time of adhesive. They can also be used to dry lashes after cleansing and rinsing. Nano misters and nebulizers are used to mist distilled water onto eyelash extensions to cure adhesive.

MIRRORS

A dental mirror is used to easily view the lashes while working behind the client's head. It helps when looking for "stickies" and ensuring there are no gaps during an eyelash extension service. A hand mirror is used to show the client the finished look.

SILICONE EYELASH LIFTING SHIELDS AND RODS

Eyelash lifting shields and rods are used during eyelash lifting (perming) services. Made of silicon, they are adhered to the eyelid using lash lift adhesive, and then the eyelashes are adhered to the shields or rods **(Figure 5–5)**. They help form the curve in the lash, so picking out the correct size is important. Most of the client's lashes should reach the half-way point of the shield or rod. If the size is too small, most of the lashes will reach the top, creating too much curl or even a crimp at the tip of the lashes. If the size is too large, there won't be enough of a curve in the lash.

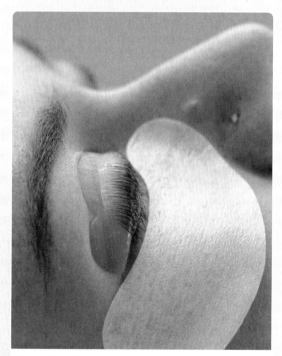

Fig. 5-5: Silicone eyelash lifting shields.

Single-Use Implements

Single-use implements, also known as *disposable implements*, are used once on a client and then discarded, preferably while the client is present. Clients notice cleanliness, and it instills confidence in their safety while in your care. The following are common disposable implements for eyelash services:

- Nitrile gloves are used for infection control and personal protection.
- Client headbands are used to protect the hair and hold it out of the way.
- Eye pads are used to protect the skin, lower lashes, and in the case of eyelash extensions act as a lash map. They are typically white, but also come in other colors to help see light-colored eyelashes better. Sensitive eye pads are available for those clients with sensitive skin.
- Medical tape is used to further protect lower lashes by being placed over eye pads; it can be used to protect a jade stone or crystal stone from adhesive residue. There is also sensitive medical tape for clients with sensitive skin.
- Mascara brushes and wands are used to comb through both eyelashes and eyebrows.
- Micro swabs are used to apply product to eyelashes or eyebrows, such as lash primer or adhesive remover. They have a lint-free and non-absorbent head that is great for precision application **(Figure 5–6)**.

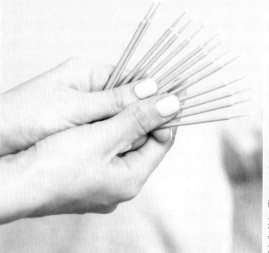

Fig. 5-6: Micro swabs.

- Lint-free applicators are used to apply product to eyelashes or eyebrows as well as cleansing eyelashes. They have a lint-free, flocked tip with a slight slant **(Figure 5-7a)**. Typically called *doe-foot applicators*, they are often used for lipstick or lip gloss application.

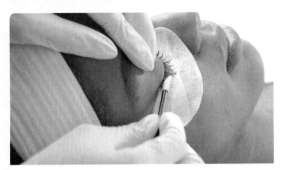

Fig. 5-7a: Lint-free applicators are used for applying eye and lip products and cleansing lashes and brows.

- Interdental brushes are used during eyebrow lamination services **(Figure 5-7b)**. Although usually used for dental purposes, they are great for brushing through eyebrow hair for precision shaping because they are smaller than mascara brushes.

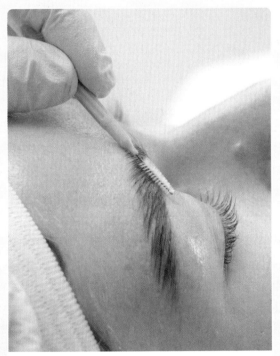

Fig. 5-7b: Interdental brushes are used during eyebrow lamination services.

- Adhesive stickers can be used on jade stones, lash tiles, or crystals to protect the surface from product residue. This makes it easier to clean up and ensures client safety.

- Eyelash cleansing brushes can be given to clients as an aftercare tool and should never be reused on another client. The brush is soft, lint-free, and designed to cleanse between the lash line and extensions to prevent debris buildup.

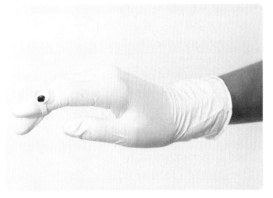

- Glue rings and glue cups are worn on the finger and act as holders for adhesive or other product while performing eyelash services. There are various styles that differ by shape, and some glue rings even have removable cups.
- Cotton pads are used to cleanse, rinse, and dry eyelashes during services.
- Y combs are used during lash lifting (perming) services. They come in the manufacturer's kits and may vary in design. Typically, they have a base to hold onto and then the tip splits into a "Y" shape **(Figure 5-8)**. One side of the tip is blunt and used to push the lashes down onto the shields or rods after application of adhesive. The other side has teeth to comb and separate the lashes.

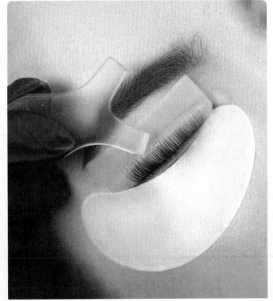

Fig. 5-8: Y comb.

Ch. 05: Tools, Products, and Ingredients

Equipment

A lash salon or treatment area must have certain equipment to properly perform eyelash and eyebrow services:

- Hydraulic table—an adjustable, comfortable table for your clients to lay or sit on.
- Technician's chair—an ergonomic, comfortable, durable, stain resistant, and easily cleaned chair for you to sit on. The idea chair has wheels for maneuverability and hydraulics for height adjustment. Some may have an adjustable back depending on preference.
- Lash cart/trolley—a rolling cart to hold products and tools while working.
- Adjustable light or magnifying light glasses—an overhead adjustable light is ideal. Technicians can also wear magnifying glasses with a light attachment.
- Autoclave—in addition to disinfecting, some states require all multiuse metal implements be sterilized in an autoclave. Check your local state licensing board on autoclave use and infection control laws.
- Trash container—a trash container with a foot-operated, self-closing lid should be located next to your lashing station. Line it with a disposable trash bag and close when not in use. Empty it at the end of each workday and clean and disinfect it often.

✓ Check In

5. What is the difference between single-use implements and multiuse tools?

6. Which tweezers are best for creating and picking up lash fans? Why?

7. Are eyelash cleansing brushes single- or multiuse implements?

Workbook Assessment

Fill in the blanks below using words from the provided word bank.

Fill in the Blank

QUESTION 3:

Tweezers are commonly made of either ...., which is usually rust resistant, or ...., which is completely rust-free.

QUESTION 4:

The .... tweezer, also called an L-shaped tweezer, has a sharply angled curved tip and is perfect for creating, as well as picking up, lash fans.

QUESTION 5:

During an eyebrow service, you are shaping a client's eyebrows. You are most likely to use a(n) .... tweezer.

QUESTION 6:

You are applying eyelash extensions to a client and working with multiple tweezers with different tips. To remove the tape and the eye pad at the end of the service, you would use a(n) .... tweezer.

QUESTION 7:

Rafaelle is performing eyelash perming for a client. They are using a tool whose tip is shaped like a sharply angled pick to separate the lashes so that they do not stick together. Rafaelle is most likely using a(n) .... tool.

QUESTION 8:

A lash .... (or lash palette) is made of acrylic, crystal, or glass and is used for organizing lash extension strips. Some lash palettes have a small well that can be used for the lash ....

Word Bank

dental
shields
jade
silicone
round
stainless steel
hand
titanium
adhesive
distilled
eyelash separation
tile
nebulizer
slant
boot tip

Ch. 05: Tools, Products, and Ingredients

QUESTION 9:

While applying eyelash extensions, the lash technician usually places the lash

.... on a(n) .... stone or a crystal to keep it cool and prevent it from drying rapidly.

QUESTION 10:

You are applying eyelash extensions to a client. The weather is dry with low humidity, which has slowed down the curing of the lash adhesive. To speed up the curing,

you must use a nano mister or a(n) .... to mist eyelash extensions with

.... water.

QUESTION 11:

While applying eyelash extensions to a client, Estevan is sitting behind the client's head. To see if there are any gaps in the lashes, Estevan is most likely to use a(n)

.... mirror. To show the finished look to the client after the service is

complete, he is most likely to use a(n) .... mirror.

QUESTION 12:

To shape lashes during eyelash lifting services, lash technicians use eyelash lifting

.... and rods, which are made from the material ....

Word Bank

dental
shields
jade
silicone
round
stainless steel
hand
titanium
adhesive
distilled
eyelash separation
tile
nebulizer
slant
boot tip

Ch. 05: Tools, Products, and Ingredients

Eyelash Extensions

 Learning Objective 04

Compare the different eyelash extension options.

In this section, you will encounter the different types of eyelash extensions available. Because eyelash extension services will always be customized based on your clients' natural eyelashes and their desired look, it is important to know the relative benefits of each eyelash extension type.

Types of Eyelash Extensions

Eyelash extensions are available in a variety of materials, from the classic mink to the modern synthetic. All these extension types have their pros and cons to consider during client consultation.

MINK

Mink lashes are controversial because they come from a live animal and, as such, are not produced as commonly as they used to be. These lashes come from a mink's tail, typically a Siberian or Chinese mink. Mink lashes are hollow inside, making them very soft, light weight, and extremely natural looking. Real mink extensions last much longer because of how light they are, allowing several to be applied per lash. Mink lashes are often referred to as luxury lashes. Typically, all mink full sets cost between $300 and $500. The lashes don't come curled, so they must be permed or curled with heat. If you choose to curl with heat instead of perm, the client will have to keep curling them at home because they will lose their curl whenever they get wet. Mink lashes generally come in a more matte or satin finish. They are prone to causing reactions and allergies because they come from a live animal.

FAUX MINK

Faux mink lashes are manmade fibers that imitate mink lashes. There are no animals used in their production, but they retain the light weight of mink fur. Unlike mink, faux mink lashes have a permanent curl and come in a wide variety of lengths, diameters, and curls.[7]

SILK

Silk lashes are typically synthetic silk fiber and not actually natural silkworm silk. Technology is always advancing, so manufacturers are now creating silk lashes that are finer and more natural looking than ever before. These are comparable to mink lashes, without the allergy risk. Silk lashes typically have a more natural look, but because they can come in different diameters you can get a somewhat more dramatic appearance by selecting a thicker lash. Silk lashes hold their curl, even if the curl is not generally as uniform as synthetic lashes. These lashes are shinier but vary brand to brand. Silk lashes are very versatile and come in different colors, finishes, curls, and lengths.

SYNTHETIC

Synthetic lash extensions are widely used and the most common type of lashes. Synthetic doesn't necessarily mean low quality; it just means that they are made from polished acrylic material, which makes them firmer and sturdier. Synthetic lashes have a glossy finish and are shinier than mink and silk lashes. These lashes are darker and thicker because of their tapered design. They come in a wide variety of thicknesses, curls, and colors. Synthetic lashes at a thicker diameter will give you the most dramatic effect; however, they feel stiffer and fall off quicker than other lash types. Long-term use of synthetic lashes can also cause damage to the natural lashes.

Eyelash Extension Curl

Eyelash extension curl ranges from straight to very curved. The different curl styles allow eyelash technicians to customize lash map designs based on eye shape as well as desired look **(Table 5-1)**. For example, if you have a client with straight lashes, J and B curls will work to create a natural lift. C and D curls create more open-eyed, dramatic looks. L curls have a flat base that can be applied to monolid and hooded eyes to create lift.

Table 5-1	Eyelash Extension Curls			
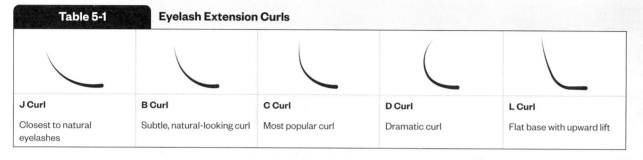				
J Curl	**B Curl**	**C Curl**	**D Curl**	**L Curl**
Closest to natural eyelashes	Subtle, natural-looking curl	Most popular curl	Dramatic curl	Flat base with upward lift

Eyelash Extension Diameter and Length

Eyelash extensions vary in width from 0.05 millimeters to 0.25 millimeters **(Figure 5-9)**. Select extensions that are the same diameter as the client's natural lash. If the client wants a more dramatic look, only choose extensions that are slightly thicker.

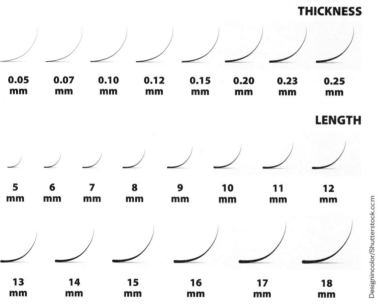

Fig. 5-9: Eyelash extension diameters and lengths.

Eyelash extension lengths range from 5 millimeters to 18 millimeters **(Figure 5-9)**. The longer the extension, the more dramatic the look. When choosing length, do not go beyond two to three millimeters longer than the client's natural lash length.

> ⚠ **Caution!**
>
> Be aware that as the width or length of the extension increases, so does the weight of the lash. The client's natural lash needs to be able to support the weight of the extensions used. This is especially important to keep in mind while creating volume lashes!

✓ Check In

8. Which lash type has the highest risk for allergic reaction?

   ....
   ....

9. If your client wants a more dramatic look, how far can you upsize lash diameter and length?

   ....
   ....

Workbook Assessment

Multiple Response

Please mark the correct answer(s) for each question. More than one answer may apply.

QUESTION 13:
Which of the following types of lash extensions is referred to as luxury lashes?

- ☐ human hair lashes
- ☐ mink lashes
- ☐ synthetic lashes
- ☐ silk lashes

QUESTION 14:
Which of the following statements are true of mink eyelash extensions?

- ☐ They have to be permed.
- ☐ They last longer as they are very light.
- ☐ They are likely to cause allergic reactions.
- ☐ They usually have a highly glossy finish.

QUESTION 15:
You have a client who wants natural looking but thick and dramatic eyelash extensions with a shiny finish. They also want the lashes to hold curl so that they do not have to curl them repeatedly. Which of the following types of eyelash extensions would you recommend to them?

- ☐ synthetic eyelash extensions
- ☐ human hair eyelash extensions
- ☐ mink eyelash extensions
- ☐ silk eyelash extensions

QUESTION 16:
Identify the true statements about synthetic lashes.

- [ ] They are made from acrylic.
- [ ] They are of inferior quality and less sturdy than other types of lash extensions.
- [ ] They have a glossy finish and are shinier than other types of lash extensions.
- [ ] They are the safest type of extensions for long-term usage.

QUESTION 17:
Which of the following types of eyelash extension curls is the closest to the natural lashes?

- [ ] D curl
- [ ] L curl
- [ ] J curl
- [ ] C curl

QUESTION 18:
You have a client with hooded eyes. The client wants a look that would minimize the droopy over crease and provide a lift to the eyes. Which of the following types of curls would you apply to achieve the client's desired look?

- [ ] L curls
- [ ] J curls
- [ ] B curls
- [ ] D curls

QUESTION 19:
You have a client who has straight eyelashes and wants eyelash extensions that will give a natural lift to the lashes. Which of the following types of lash curls can you use to create the desired look?

- [ ] J curls
- [ ] B curls
- [ ] C curls
- [ ] D curls

QUESTION 20:
What is the most popular eyelash extension curl?

- [ ] J curl
- [ ] D curl
- [ ] B curl
- [ ] C curl

QUESTION 21:
A client, whose eyelashes are 0.10 millimeters thick, wants dramatic eyelash extensions. Which of the following options would you recommend?

- [ ] 0.13-millimeter-thick extensions
- [ ] 0.07-millimeter-thick extensions
- [ ] 0.25-millimeter-thick extensions
- [ ] 0.10-millimeter-thick extensions

QUESTION 22:
For a client with 8-millimeter-long lashes, which length of eyelash extensions is the most suitable?

- [ ] 6 millimeters
- [ ] 15 to 18 millimeters
- [ ] 10 to 11 millimeters
- [ ] 12 to 15 millimeters

Service Products and Ingredients

> **Learning Objective 05**
>
> **Recognize the professional products used during an eyelash or eyebrow service.**

Spend time familiarizing yourself with each professional product used during eyelash and eyebrow services, what chemicals they contain, and what they do. You must also know how to properly store these products and remove them from their containers in a hygienic manner.

> **Caution!**
>
> Check with your state board if lash lifts, tints, and brow laminations can be performed under your license as it varies from state to state.

Eyelash Cleanser

One of the most important steps in eyelash extension services and aftercare is cleansing the eyelashes of dirt, oil, makeup, and debris. Eyelash cleanser is specially formulated to cleanse without affecting the eyelash extension adhesive. A quality cleanser will not leave residue on the eyelashes. It is not like a regular facial cleanser or makeup remover, which could either strip the lashes of too much moisture or leave a film. Either of these will compromise lash retention and therefore client satisfaction.

When selecting an eyelash cleanser, avoid those with:

- Oil (including mineral oil and all aliases)
- Glycol
- Sulfates and surfactants
- Parabens
- Triclosan
- Salts[8]

> **Caution!**
>
> Be wary of homemade lash cleanser formulas as most contain baby shampoo, which is not advised for the eye area.

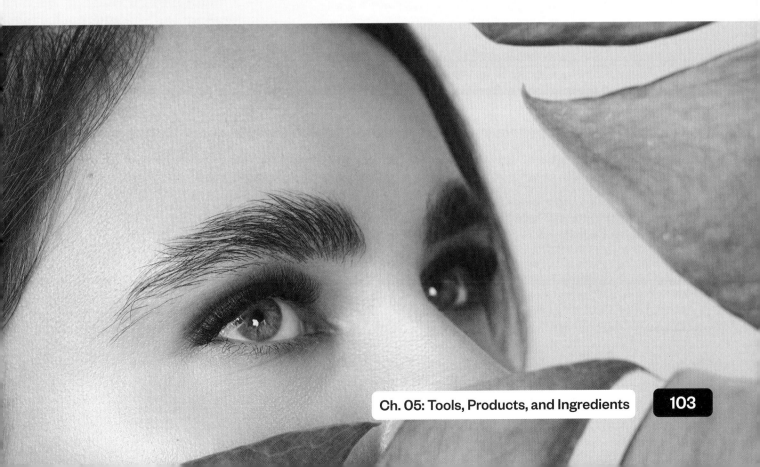

Eyelash Extension Products

On top of adhesive and extensions themselves, primer and adhesive remover are important products for eyelash extension services.

PRIMER

Application of eyelash extension primer is an optional step when performing eyelash extension services. Eyelash extension primer is made from three key ingredients: dimethyl ketone (acetone), polyethanol (alcohol), and water.[9] It is designed to remove any oils present on the natural lashes, which helps optimize adhesion of the eyelash extension and ultimately retention **(Figure 5-10)**. When applying, be sure not to touch the client's skin as this can cause a burning sensation.

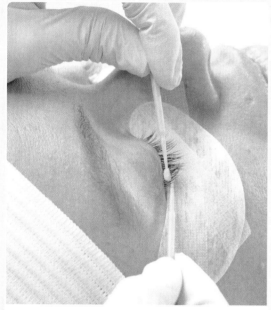

Fig. 5-10: Apply primer to lashes with micro swabs or lint-free applicators.

ADHESIVE REMOVER

Adhesive remover is required to safely remove eyelash extensions. Eyelash extension adhesive remover is formulated to break down the bonds of the adhesive so that the eyelash extension breaks free from the natural lash. Adhesive removers come in cream and gel formulas that are designed to sit on the lashes without getting into the eyes. After the adhesive remover has been allowed to process according to the manufacturer's guidelines, extensions should be able to be swiped off. Be careful that adhesive remover never enters the client's eyes.

Lifting and Lamination Products

Eyelash lifting and eyebrow lamination have several unique products, including chemical solutions for lifting and neutralization.

LASH LIFT ADHESIVE

Lash lift adhesive is used during eyelash lifting (perming) services. It is used to secure shields or rods to the client's eyelid as well as to secure the client's natural lashes to the shields or rods. It is easily dissolved using water.

LIFTING SOLUTION

Lifting solution is used in eyelash lifting services and eyebrow lamination services and found in their accompanying kits. Thioglycolic acid, polyacrylamide, propylene glycol methyl paraben, purified water, and monoethanolamide are some of the ingredients included in lifting solutions. As the solution processes, it breaks down the bonds of the hairs. In the case of eyelash lifting, it allows the lashes to form to the shield or rod. For eyebrows, it allows the hairs to relax into the shape they were brushed. Lash or eyebrow hair may become damaged or brittle if solution is left on too long, so always be sure to follow the manufacturer's recommended processing time. When removing the solution, always follow the manufacturer's directions as to whether it needs wet, dry, or a combination removal.

 Caution!

Never use hair perming solution as an eyelash or eyebrow lifting solution! Only use the solutions in kits designated specifically for eyelashes or eyebrows.

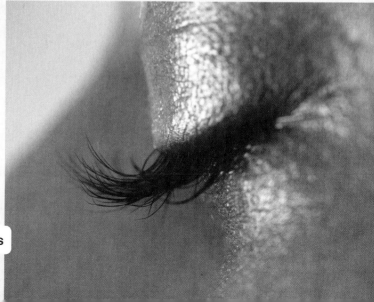

NEUTRALIZING SOLUTION

Neutralizing solution is used in eyelash lifting services and eyebrow lamination services and found in their accompanying kits. Sodium bromate, polyacrylamide, polysorbate, purified water, propylene glycol, and methyl paraben are ingredients that comprise neutralizing solution. As the solution processes, it reforms the bonds of the hairs. In eyelash lifting, it sets the lashes into the shape of the shields or rods **(Figure 5–11)**. In brow lamination, the brow hairs reform into the shape they are brushed. As with lifting solution, always be sure to follow the manufacturer's recommended processing time and removal method to avoid damaging lash or brow hairs.

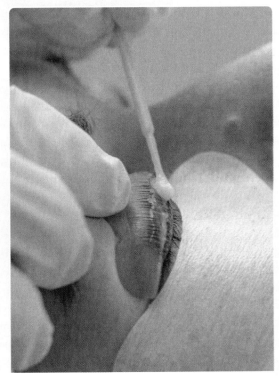

Fig. 5-11: Neutralizing solution reforms lashes into the curve of the shields or rods.

 Here's a Tip

When applying lifting and neutralizing solutions to eyelashes, apply only to the middle section of the lashes and never the tips or base. By following this guideline, you will avoid both overprocessing the tips and getting the solution in the client's eyes.

POST-TREATMENT LOTION

Post-treatment lotion is an optional product used in eyelash lifting services and eyebrow lamination services and found in their accompanying kits. It is used to nourish lash or brow hairs. Follow manufacturer's direction on processing time and removal. This lotion is applied using micro swabs or lint-free applicators.

Eyelash and Brow Tints

Eyelash and eyebrow tints are found in their respective kits. They are used to darken the eyelash or eyebrow hair. Should you need to replace only the developer instead of an entire kit, be sure to replace with the appropriate percentage of developer. Check with your manufacturer on the proper developer percentage. Although some tints contain synthetic coal tar, the main ingredient for eyelash tinting formula is phenylenediamine (PPD), a chemical chosen because it can be washed without running. PPD is a chemical also found in temporary tattoos, printing ink, and some gases. Phenylenediamine requires oxygen to activate, so hydrogen peroxide is added during processing. When the two mix, the solution begins to oxidize. If at any time during the service the client complains of irritating, itching, or burning sensations, the tint must be removed immediately. Flushing the eyes with cold or tepid water is recommended. Severe reactions can appear as red, swollen, and sometimes blistered skin.

 Check In

10. What is it called when a chemical changes because of the addition of oxygen?

11. What does lifting solution do as it processes?

12. How is eyelash cleanser unlike regular facial cleanser or makeup remover?

Ch. 05: Tools, Products, and Ingredients

Workbook Assessment

Fill in the blanks below using words from the provided word bank.

Fill in the Blank

QUESTION 23:

After applying eyelash extensions to a client, Kai advises the client to use only

eyelash .... to remove dirt or makeup from the eyelashes as it does not adversely affect the eyelash extension adhesive.

QUESTION 24:

The key ingredients in eyelash extension .... are dimethyl ketone, polyethanol, and water.

QUESTION 25:

Brenna is performing an eyelash refill service for a client. Using a micro swab, she applies a product to the old overgrown lash extensions and waits for 5 minutes. She then swipes off the extensions, which easily detach from the natural lashes. In the

given scenario, Brenna has used the micro swab to apply a(n) .... to the lash extensions.

QUESTION 26:

Eyelash extension primer removes .... that are present on the natural

lashes. This improves adhesion as well as .... of eyelash extensions.

QUESTION 27:

When performing a lash perm service for a client, a lash technician must adhere

lash lift shields or rods to the .... of the client with a(n) .... adhesive.

QUESTION 28:

.... solution is used in eyelash perming services and eyebrow

.... services to break down the bonds of the hairs.

Word Bank

lifting
micro swab
lifting solution
phenylenediamine
post-treatment
primer
lamination
adhesive remover
cleanser
eyelid(s)
oils
oxygen
neutralizing solution
lash lift
retention

Ch. 05: Tools, Products, and Ingredients

QUESTION 29:

In eyelash lifting, the .... sets the curl of the eyelashes in the desired shape.

QUESTION 30:

The .... breaks down the bonds of the lash hairs, whereas the

.... forms those bonds again.

QUESTION 31:

After completing eyebrow lamination services for a client, Chen prefers to apply a(n)

...................., lotion to the client's eyebrows to nourish them. Chen most likely

uses either a(n) ...., or a lint-free applicator to apply it.

QUESTION 32:

The main ingredient in eyebrow and eyelash tints is the chemical ....,

(PPD), which is activated by the gas ....

Chapter Glossary

Term	Page	Definition
boot tip tweezer *boot tip **TWEE**-zur*	p. 092	also called *L-shaped tweezer*; has a sharply angled curved tip and is mainly used for volume and mega volume lashing
carbon black ***KAAR**-bun blak*	p. 088	dark black powder used as a pigment; used as a coloring agent in adhesives
curved tweezer *kurvd **TWEE**-zur*	p. 092	has a gentle curved tip and is typically used for isolation as well as precision placement of lash extensions
cyanoacrylate *sy-ah-noh-**AK**-ruh-layt*	p. 087	main component of eyelash extension adhesives; an acrylate monomer that is cured and used as an adhesive
formaldehyde *fr-**MAL**-duh-hide*	p. 088	colorless gas with a strong odor; a byproduct of curing cyanoacrylates
hydroquinone *hai-drow-kwuh-**NOWN***	p. 088	used as a stabilizing agent; keeps cyanoacrylate from curing in the bottle by stopping the polymerization process
polymerization ***PAHL**-uh-muh-ry-**ZAY**-shuhn*	p. 088	chemical process through which monomers form bonds with water to create long molecular chains; for example, cyanoacrylate turning from liquid adhesive into a solid glue
polymethyl methacrylate (PMMA) ***PAA**-lee-meh-thl muh-**THA**-kruh-layt*	p. 088	used as a thickening agent; a synthetic resin produced from the polymerization of methyl methacrylate
round tweezers *rownd **TWEE**-zurs*	p. 092	have rounded tips that make it ideal for safely removing tape and eye pads after a service is completed
slant tweezers *slant **TWEE**-zurs*	p. 092	typically used for eyebrow shaping; however, can also be used for applying temporary strip or cluster eyelashes
straight tweezers *strayt **TWEE**-zurs*	p. 092	long and narrow, ending in a tapered point ideal for picking up and placing lash extensions

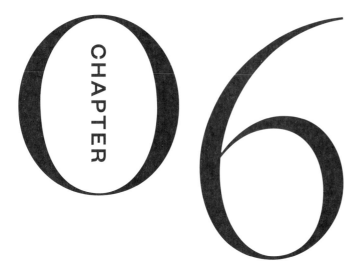

Eyelash Extension Application

🚩 Learning Objectives

After completing this chapter, you will be able to:

1. Explain why knowledge of eyelash extension application is essential to eyelash extension technicians.
2. Demonstrate a thorough client consultation for eyelash extensions.
3. Summarize how to choose the appropriate length and thickness of extension to best suit your client.
4. Describe the purpose of a lash map.
5. Recognize the conditions that contraindicate eyelash services.
6. Discuss how to prepare the client for lash application.
7. Apply temporary cluster or strip lashes to the client safely.
8. Perform a classic eyelash application.
9. Perform a volume eyelash application.
10. Perform an eyelash refill procedure.
11. Perform an eyelash extension removal service.
12. Describe aftercare instructions for eyelash extension clients.
13. Identify solutions to common eyelash extension problems.

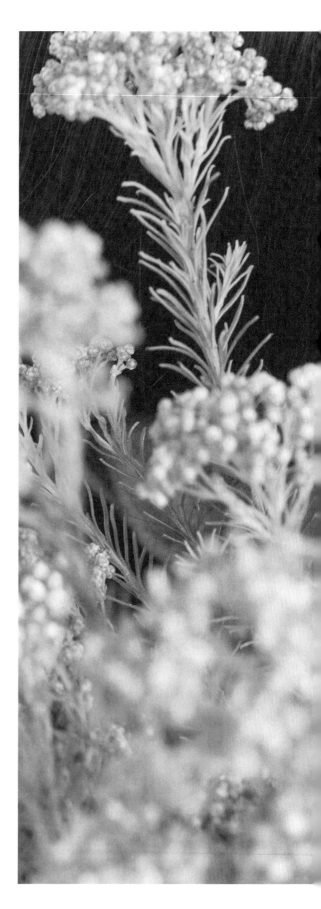

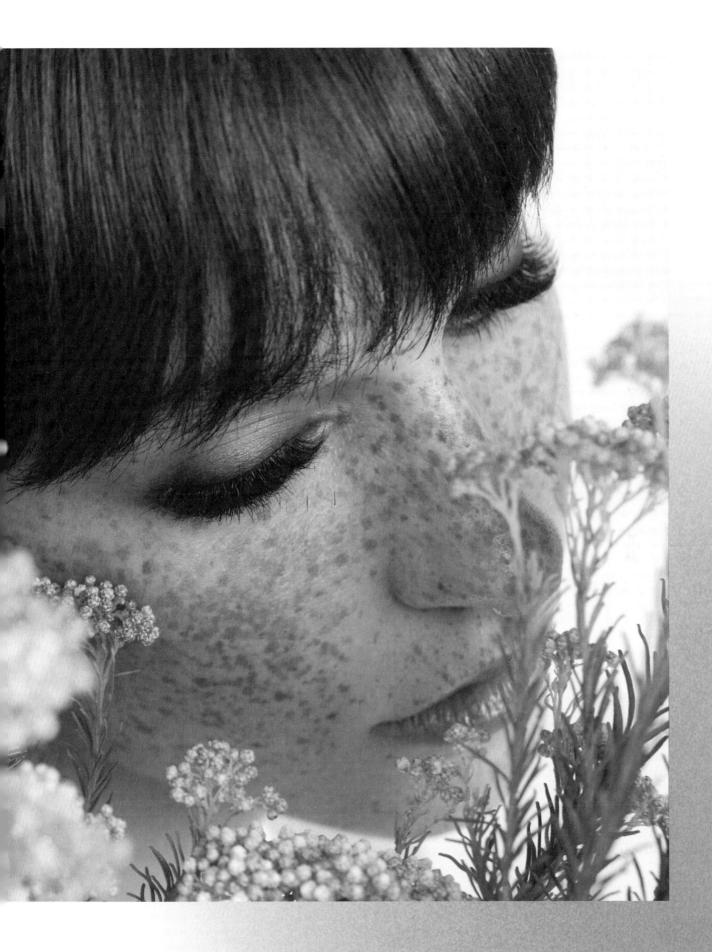

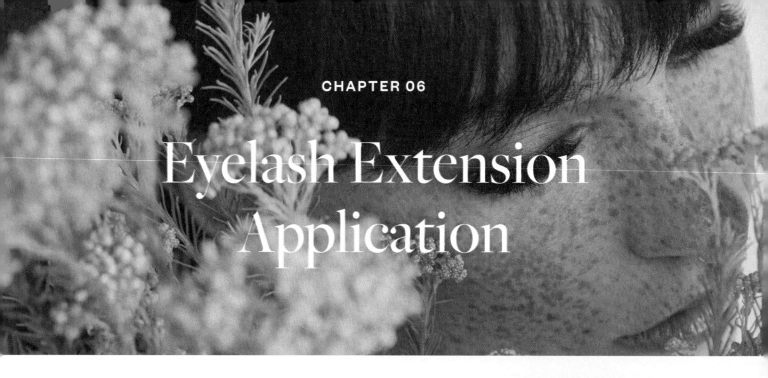

CHAPTER 06

Eyelash Extension Application

Why Study Eyelash Extension Application?

 Learning Objective 01

Explain why knowledge of eyelash extension application is essential to eyelash extension technicians.

Eyelash extensions are one of the most lucrative services you can offer in the beauty industry, with low overhead and high-ticketed bookings. Being able to apply, refill, and remove lash extensions correctly, efficiently, and safely are the skills needed to succeed in a market where both demand and client expectations are high. It is important to keep in mind that this is not a one-size-fits-all service. Just as everyone's eyelashes, eyes, and face are unique, so too should every client's eyelash extension application service be customized to fit their needs. Eyelash technicians must also teach the client how to care for their extensions—eyelash extensions can be enjoyed year-round by following simple maintenance and care instructions along with retouch applications.

Eyelash technicians should study and have a thorough understanding of eyelash extension application because:

- The client consultation is the time to ensure the service provided will be safe, comfortable, long-lasting, and flattering to the client's desires and facial features.
- Accurate and efficient application of classic and volume lashes, as well as filling and removing them, is the beating heart of the eyelash technician's job.
- Temporary lashes offer a shorter term, affordable alternative that fits the needs of some clients better than full eyelash extensions.
- Properly preparing the client before their lash service and sending them off with good aftercare instructions are both key to increasing retention and satisfaction.
- Being able to troubleshoot client issues and their own performance can only help eyelash technicians improve over the life of their career.

Check In

1. Why do you think it is important to study eyelash extension application?

....

....

Client Consultation

Learning Objective 02

Demonstrate a thorough client consultation for eyelash extensions.

The eyes are one of the most delicate and sensitive areas of the face. The eyes will react to sensitivities and allergies more quickly than any other area of the face. Proper consultation is critical for a successful lash application. Ask clients to come in prior to their lash-application appointment for a 15-minute consultation to discuss what they should expect during the procedure. Examine the eye area: If there is visible redness, swelling, itching, or crusting, do not perform the lash application. Instead, refer the client to a physician or eye doctor to determine the cause. The condition should be cleared before you apply the lashes.

Some adhesives may have fumes that can cause a burning sensation to the eyes. During your consultation, you will be able to determine if sensitivity may be an issue for your client. If sensitivity seems likely, perform a patch test at least 24 hours before the application (but preferably 48 hours to give you time to reschedule). At the application appointment, you can check for reaction. Always perform a patch test for new clients. The amount of adhesive used for the patch test is very minimal. If your client does not have a sensitivity reaction during the patch test process, this does not mean that they will not react when receiving extensions themselves. Maintain clear communication with your client so that they are aware of all risks involved with getting their lashes done.

It is important to explain to your client how to prepare for the lash appointment. Things to mention when preparing your client are:

- Prepare to lay down for over 3 hours.
- Avoid caffeine prior to the appointment, as well as nicotine, which can cause the eyes to flutter.
- Arrive with no makeup on, especially eye makeup, as this can cause poor retention.
- Prepare to keep your eyes closed for the entirety of the appointment. This also means hours of phone-free time.
- Shower prior to the appointment. It is recommended that lashes stay dry for the first 24 hours.

The consultation is the time to discuss the client's desired outcome. Will they be attending a special occasion? Do they like a more natural or dramatic look? Do they have any inspiration photos? This will help you determine what lash extension lengths will be necessary. It is also the place to set expectations with your client as to what is possible and healthy for their natural lashes. Have open communication and suggest something healthier if your client pushes for lashes they can't safely support. This will prevent an unhappy client and miscommunication on the day of the service.

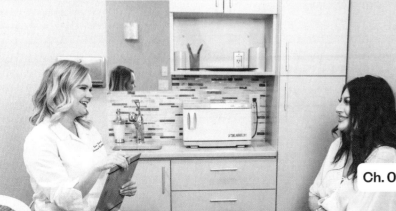

Ch. 06: Eyelash Extension Application

Consultation Forms

Your consultations will likely begin with the client filling out a consultation form or questionnaire that gathers contact information, service expectations, product use, and medical details pertaining to eye conditions and allergies or sensitivities **(Table 6–1)**. This form may also set forth the liability limits of you and your salon. It is important to go over the client consultation form and ask the client to initial that they acknowledge the risks involved and that they understand the importance of following precise instructions for aftercare given by their lash artist. Have a lawyer draft a separate consent form for you covering all liabilities in case of emergency if this information is not included in the consultation form.

Here's a Tip

Use the client consultation visit as an opportunity to discuss aftercare, offer additional services, sell retail products, and book refill services.

Table 6-1   Sample Client Consultation Form

Confidential Eyelash and Eyebrow Treatment Questionnaire

Today's Date: _____

First Name: _____ Last Name: _____ Birthday _____

Street _____ Apt# ____ City _____ State _____ Zip _____

Phone: ( ) _____ E-mail: _____

Referred by (circle one):   Friend   Social Media   Walk-In   Gift Certificate   Internet Search   Other: _____

Have you ever had an eyelash or eyebrow service ☐ Yes ☐ No

If yes, which service and what did you like (dislike) about the session?
_____

Did you experience any negative reactions (allergic/sensitivity) after the eyelash or eyebrow service? ☐ Yes ☐ No

If yes, please provide as many details as possible: _____

What are some of your goals today?
_____

Do you wear contact lenses? ☐ Yes ☐ No   If yes, are they: ☐ Hard ☐ Soft

Do you take any medications that cause your eyes to be dry or itch? ☐ Yes ☐ No

If yes, what? _____

Are you currently taking prescription drugs that affect your skin or have you taken any in the past? ☐ Yes ☐ No

If yes, describe the course and length of treatment. _____

Do you have any health condition that may cause sensitivity to your skin or eye area? ☐ Yes ☐ No

If yes, what? _____

Do you have any allergies? ☐ Yes ☐ No   If yes, please indicate. _____

Do you have any allergies to skin care products? ☐ Yes ☐ No   If yes, what? _____

I fully acknowledge that I do not have any known allergies to makeup products, or contagious conditions, or have listed them above.

Signature: _____ Date: _____

Once your client has completed the consultation form, you can start making notes on client preferences, such as length and diameter of the lash extensions to be used. A client chart is a great place for these notes **(Table 6-2)**. Write down the eyelash map so you can reference it at later appointments and adjust as the client prefers. Mark the types of products you use and what aftercare products the client takes home.

Table 6-2 — **Sample Lash Client Chart**

Name: _____ Date: _____

Service Type: Full Set | Refill

Set Type: Classic | Volume

Style: _____

Eyelash Map:

Diameter: _____ Curl: _____ Fan Volume: _____

Adhesive: _____

Tape: _____

Aftercare Products:
_____

Other Notes:
_____

Focus On

The Lash Consultation Area

The lash consultation area is the same area where you will be providing lash services. The client will need to lay down on your recliner or table to ensure you can get an accurate look at their natural lashes. Make sure that your lash station is clean, tidy, and well-lit prior to bringing your client back for a consultation. Be sure to have tools ready to perform a lash examination and patch test.

Ultimately, you will need to use your best discretion when determining if the client is a good candidate for lash extensions. Pay attention to any contraindications that present themselves. If your client's lashes are brittle, frail, or not in good health, be comfortable with turning the client away for their own safety. Suggest an alternative service, or clearly communicate why services cannot be performed.

Caution!

If your client is pregnant, be sure to mark down that the table will need to be inclined during the procedure. Provide the client an estimated procedure time so that they are prepared.

Ch. 06: Eyelash Extension Application

Check In

2. What is the appropriate action to take if a client has an unrealistic expectation of their desired lash look?

....
....

3. What is the purpose of having your client sign a consent form in addition to filling out a consultation form?

....
....

Workbook Assessment

Select whether the statements below are true or false.

True or False

QUESTION 1:
During consultation, eyelash technicians must inform clients that the eyelash extension application service can take over 3 hours.

T   F   why?...

QUESTION 2:
Saki has an eyelash extension client who has a very busy work schedule. The client is finding it difficult to find a window of 3 hours to get the lash extensions. In the given scenario, Saki can advise the client to check their emails over phone and complete some work during the wait times between different eyelash processes.

T   F   why?...

QUESTION 3:
Application of eye makeup prior to eyelash extension application can lead to poor extension retention.

T   F   why?...

QUESTION 4:
Matías, an eyelash technician, has a new eyelash extension client who arrives with a fresh cup of coffee. Matías must advise the client to avoid caffeine before the appointment as it could interfere with the results of the service.

T   F   why?...

QUESTION 5:
It is advisable for a client to avoid showering before an eyelash extension appointment.

T   F   why?...

QUESTION 6:
During consultation, a client insists on getting extensions that might harm their natural lashes. You have suggested a better, heathier alternative, but the client insists on what they want. The best practice in such cases is to agree to provide the service if the client signs a consent form and waives liability.

T   F   why?...

Choosing the Proper Extension

 Learning Objective 03

Summarize how to choose the appropriate length and thickness of extension to best suit your client.

Synthetic black lashes are the most common extensions used; however, many manufacturers carry lash extensions in a variety of colors for different occasions, events, and client requests. Lash lengths and thicknesses will vary depending on what the client's natural lashes can hold. Keep in mind to never exceed double the length or thickness of the natural lash to prevent permanent damage to the follicle. You should also always strive to tailor your client's lashes to flatter their facial features. Refer to Chapter 2, Eye and Eyelash Anatomy and Physiology, for tips on how to best suit different eye shapes, eye spacings, and face shapes.

 Here's a Tip

Hold the lash extension next to the client's natural lashes to determine if it is the appropriate weight. Do this prior to dipping the lash into adhesive.

Before considering the use and placement of variations of lash lengths, become proficient in basic lash selection and application techniques. Check the client's natural lash length and then select lashes based on the goal for the finished look.

- **Natural.** Select lashes slightly longer than the client's lashes. This makes the lashes appear fuller (**Figure 6–1**).

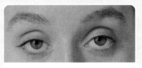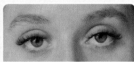

Fig. 6-1: Natural eyelashes (left) compared to a natural eyelash extension look (right).

- **Feminine.** Select lashes about a third longer than the client's lashes. If the length/diameter of the natural lash allows, increase the diameter to .20 mm for thickness and flair slightly longer at outside corners.

- **Dramatic/maximum.** Select lashes one and a half times the length of the client's lashes. If the natural lash allows, use .20 to .25 mm diameter for thickness and effect.

Keep in mind the growth cycles that all hair goes through. Hair in the anagen phase is too fragile to lash. Hair in the catagen phase is healthy and strong, and has the most color of the growth cycles. This is the ideal lashing phase. Hair in the telogen phase is no longer growing, but still attached. Applying a lash extension to a hair in the telogen phase is useless as the natural lash will soon shed. Explain to your client that all hair falls out, and shedding is common. Always set and maintain client expectations around the lash extension service.

Types of Lashes

Lashes come in a variation of *classic* and *volume* lashes. Classic lashes are meant to be placed at a 1:1 ratio. What this means is that one single lash extension is placed on one single natural lash. Classic lashes are typically heavier in weight and diameter. Classic lashes should never be utilized as volume lashes. This is detrimental to the natural lash health and would be far too heavy. Volume lashes are much lighter in weight and are formed into a fan using multiple lashes to create a fuller/thicker look. The number of lashes used in a fan is determined by the lash technician based on the client's natural lash health and desired outcome. Classic lashing is considered beginners lashing and should always be mastered first. Volume lashing is an advanced technique and cannot be completed correctly without the knowledge of classic basics. The two styles can be combined to create a *hybrid* set of lashes. Depending on the client's desired look, you can customize the set with equal parts classic and volume, or more of one or the other.

✓ Check In

4. What are the limits on length and thickness when it comes to selecting lash extensions?

   ....

   ....

   ....

5. What is the difference between classic and volume lashes?

   ....

   ....

   ....

   ....

Workbook Assessment

Multiple Response

Please mark the correct answer(s) for each question. More than one answer may apply.

QUESTION 7:
The natural lashes' ability to hold extensions is the basis to decide what?

- ☐ the length and thickness of the lash extensions
- ☐ the curl of the lash extensions
- ☐ whether to use silk or synthetic lash extensions
- ☐ the lash map

QUESTION 8:
Why should you never apply lash extensions that are double the length of the natural lashes?

- ☐ They look awkward.
- ☐ They can damage the natural lash.
- ☐ They are more likely to clump together.
- ☐ They require special aftercare that requires multiple visits.

QUESTION 9:

For a client who wants a natural look, you must select lash extensions that are what?

- [ ] the same length as the client's natural lashes
- [ ] half as long as the client's natural lashes
- [ ] about a third longer than the client's natural lashes
- [ ] slightly longer than the client's natural lashes

QUESTION 10:

Which of the following is a feature of the lashes that creates a feminine look?

- [ ] The lashes at the outer corners of the eye are slightly longer.
- [ ] The longest lashes are at the inner corner of the eye.
- [ ] The longest lashes are at the middle of the lash line.
- [ ] The longer lashes are placed throughout the set to form "spikes."

QUESTION 11:

What is the recommended diameter of lash extensions to create a feminine look?

- [ ] 0.25 mm
- [ ] 0.15 mm
- [ ] 0.20 mm
- [ ] 0.10 mm

QUESTION 12:

Andrei has a client who wants their lash extensions to give them a dramatic look. The client's natural lashes are 10 mm long. Which of the following combinations of extension length and thickness should Andrei recommend to them?

- [ ] 12 mm long and 0.20 mm thick
- [ ] 15 mm long and 0.25 mm thick
- [ ] 20 mm long and 0.25 mm thick
- [ ] 10 mm long and 0.25 mm thick

QUESTION 13:

Which of the following statements are true of eyelash hairs in the catagen phase?

- [ ] They are ideal for lash application.
- [ ] They have the most color of all the growth stages.
- [ ] They are strong and heathy.
- [ ] They are still growing.

QUESTION 14:

In which of the following growth stages is it useless to apply extensions?

- [ ] the anagen restart stage
- [ ] the anagen stage
- [ ] the catagen stage
- [ ] the telogen stage

QUESTION 15:

Which of the following statements are true of classic lash extensions?

- [ ] They can be combined with volume lashes to create a hybrid set.
- [ ] They are lighter than volume lashes.
- [ ] They can be used as single or volume lashes.
- [ ] They are good for new lash technicians as they are relatively easier to apply.

QUESTION 16:

Santana is creating a lash map for a client. The client wants full volume lashes. Which of the following should Santana take into consideration to decide the number of lashes in lash fans?

- [ ] the health of the client's natural lashes
- [ ] the client's schedule
- [ ] the client's desired outcome
- [ ] the length of client's natural lash

Ch. 06: Eyelash Extension Application

Eyelash Mapping

 Learning Objective 04

Describe the purpose of a lash map.

Making a lash map is the key to creating seamless sets that accentuate a client's unique features. No two sets will or should ever be the same, as everyone has unique features. It is important that you take this into consideration and avoid thinking of lashes as a "one-size-fits-all" service.

What Is a Lash Map?

A **lash map** is a guide for placing specific lengths of lash extensions in a set. This plan will dictate how the lash extensions will look upon opening the eye. While making a lash map, take into consideration the natural shape of the eye, the distance between the lash line and eyebrow, the length and thickness of the natural lash, and the client's desired outcome. Note that your main priority as a technician is to maintain the integrity of the client's natural lashes. Any style that could be damaging to the natural lashes should not be completed.

While lash mapping, note that placement of the longest extension determines what will be accentuated. For example, if the longest length is placed in the middle of the eye, the eye will appear larger and more open. If the length is placed on the outer corner, it can give the illusion that the eyes are smaller, as the eyes appear slender and drawn upward. The length of the extensions should never go above the eyebrow. Take into consideration how much space is between the client's lash line and brow. Default to a shorter lash if necessary.

If the client presents with short natural lashes, a long length will not be suitable for them. The only suitable option for short, fine texture natural lashes is to place a shorter/smaller diameter extension to maintain the health of their natural lashes. Placing a longer/larger diameter lash will cause damage to the follicle and potentially permanent hair loss.

Make a lash map at the beginning of every full set and the beginning of every fill. This is imperative to the symmetry and consistency of each eye. During an eyelash extension service, you will draw the lash map with a felt-tipped marker onto the gel eye pads after applying them to the client. You will draw lines to create sections. Within those sections, write down the length needed for each section.

Types of Lash Maps

When crafting a look for clients, you can use different types of maps to create a certain look based on the client consultation. Ensure the client will be happy with the final look by describing the different styles and if possible, have pictures available. Please note that there are many lash maps; the options to follow are three common styles.

OPEN-EYE LASH MAP

An *open-eye lash map* tries to give the illusion that the eyes are wider and more open than they appear. This map is most suitable for clients with smaller eyes, clients with hooded eyes, or clients who do not want lashes that look too dramatic. The longest length of the map should be directly in the middle of the eye, tapering down on the inner and outer corners **(Figure 6–2)**.

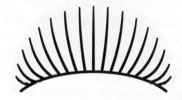

Fig. 6-2: Open-eye lash map.

TEXTURED LASH MAP

The goal of a *textured lash map* is that the lashes appear wispy and natural when the client opens their eyes. This map is suitable for any client and will compliment any eye shape. It appeals to clients who do not like the uniform lash look. This map is one of the tougher styles to accomplish because the different length extensions create a texture and depth that resembles the natural lash growth cycle. There is a lot of room for creativity and personalization during these sets. With a textured set, you will make a lash map in the uniform manner and place longer "spikes" throughout the set **(Figure 6–3)**. These spikes should be 2 to 3 mm longer than the length that would be there in a uniform lash map. The more spikes, the more textured the set will be.

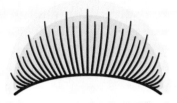

Fig. 6-3: Textured lash map.

 Focus On

Lush and Glam Lash Map

The "spike" technique can be used to create a thick, lush, glamorous look. For this map, use long lash extensions evenly across the eye. Then, place a longer lash extension for every second or third lash—alternating 12 mm/14 mm, for example. This lash map really flaunts the attention-grabbing texture. Although you are using long lashes across the eye, always remember to never exceed double the length of the natural lash.

CAT-EYE LASH MAP

A *cat-eye lash map* aims to give the illusion that the eye is smaller and more almond shaped. This sleek look is not for everyone. This map is most suitable for clients with larger eyes, round eyes, or protruding eyes. The longest length of this map will be on the outer corners, with the shorter lengths tapering down on the inner corner **(Figure 6–4)**.

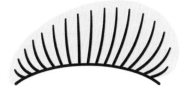

Fig. 6-4: Cat-eye lash map.

 Did You Know?

Similar to the cat-eye lash map, the *squirrel-eye lash map* uses the longest lash extension near the arch of the eyebrow or about two-thirds of the way to the outer corner of the eye. The extension lengths then taper back down to the outer edge of the eye.

How to Determine Which Map Will Suit Your Client

During the consultation, assess your client's eye shape while they are sitting upright in front of you. Speak to them about their goals, their eye shape, their face shape, and what their natural lashes can handle. Overcommunicate what you can provide so that expectations are set and known. If possible, have pictures available of what you will be providing in this service. Once you and your client have come to an agreement, proceed with the appropriate map. See Chapter 2, Eye and Eyelash Anatomy and Physiology, for more on working with differences in eye shape, eye spacing, and face shape.

Ch. 06: Eyelash Extension Application

Check In

6. What should be taken into consideration when making a lash map?

7. What will be the result if the longest length extension is placed in the middle of the eye?

Workbook Assessment

Fill in the Blank

Fill in the blanks below using words from the provided word bank.

QUESTION 17:

Bao's client wants extensions that will make her eyes look smaller and more almond shaped. To create that look, Bao must first create a diagram called a(n) ……………………, which shows the placement of different lengths of lash extensions she must use.

QUESTION 18:

In a lash map, the part that is accentuated is the one with the ………………… extensions.

QUESTION 19:

You have a client who has small eyes that are slightly hooded. In the context of types of lash maps, a(n) ……………… lash map will make the client's eyes appear more open and wider. In this style, the longest eyelashes are placed in the ………………… of the eye.

Word Bank

squirrel-eye
middle
inner
lush and glam
cat's eye
lash map
outer
open eye
follicle
spikes
textured
longest

QUESTION 20:

For a client who does not like the uniform look of eyelashes, you can recommend a(n) .... lash map. This style makes the eyelashes look wispy and natural when the client opens their eyes. The distinguishing feature of this style are the

................., which are formed by extensions that are 2 to 3 mm longer than the length of the extensions in a uniform set.

QUESTION 21:

A .... lash map uses long extensions evenly across the eye with every second or third lash longer than the rest of the lash extensions.

QUESTION 22:

Mishka has eyelash extensions that minimize his protruding eyes, making them look almond shaped. In the context of lash map styles, Mishka's lash extensions are most

likely based on the .... lash map. This means that the longest lashes are

on the .... corner of the eye and the shorter lengths taper toward the

.... corner of the eye.

QUESTION 23:

Mauna's eyelash extensions are longest where their eyebrows arch. The extension lengths then taper to smaller lengths toward the outer corner. In the context of lash

map styles, Mauna's lash extensions have a(n) .... lash map.

QUESTION 24:

If a client has short and weak natural lashes, placing a long extension is likely to

cause damage to the eyelash hair .... and may lead to permanent lash loss.

Contraindications

Learning Objective 05

Recognize the conditions that contraindicate eyelash services.

Due to the sensitivity of the eye area and the importance of eye health, there are some situations in which eyelash extensions should not be applied because they could cause harm to the client. These are known as **contraindications**. Never apply lash extensions to clients with the following conditions:

- Eye irritations, infections, allergies, or mites
- Blepharitis
- **Glaucoma**, a disease in which the optic nerve is damaged and can lead to progressive, irreversible loss of vision
- Excessive tears or persistently dry eyes

Here's a Tip

If your client experiences dry eyes, or regularly uses eye drops, lash extensions may not be for them. Consistently using an eye drop can result in poor retention. Dry eyes can be very irritating alone, and the client can experience more eye irritation with the fumes of lash extension adhesive!

- Thyroid problems affecting lash growth or causing hair loss
- Alopecia
- Recent dermal fillers, Botox injections, permanent makeup, or eye surgery
- Chemotherapy treatments, due to hair loss and increased irritation from adhesive fumes

Did You Know?

For clients undergoing chemotherapy, as an alternative to eyelash extensions show them how to simulate a lash line using eyeliner while they wait for their natural lashes to grow back. Eyelash regrowth takes roughly 56 days.

Claustrophobic clients should be aware that their eyes will remain closed for the entirety of the service. For their safety, there is no way around this. Communicate to the client what to expect and let them decide if the service will be a good fit for them based on their needs.

Clients who wear contact lenses can still receive lash extensions but will need to remove the lenses for the service. Clients should bring a pair of glasses to lash application appointments. The eyes may be a bit irritated immediately following the procedure. Wearing glasses home will give the delicate eye area a chance to adjust to the lash extensions. Always ask clients if they are regular glasses wearers. If they are, customize their set of lashes to ensure the lashes don't touch the glasses when they blink.

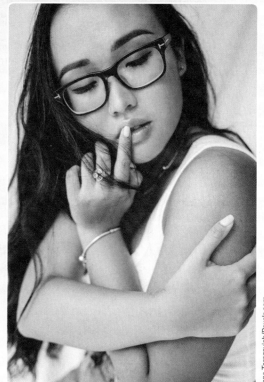

Check In

8. Name three contraindications of lash extensions.

   ....
   ....

Workbook Assessment

Multiple Choice

Please circle the correct answer for each question below.

Marisol has been a lash technician for 8 years. During this time, Marisol has experienced different kinds of cases and contraindications to lash extension. In her salon, she is the resident expert on contraindication, and all her colleagues come to her for advice.

QUESTION 25:

Marisol is most likely to tell a client that they cannot receive eyelash extensions for which of the following reasons?

A) They wear eyeglasses.

B) They use contact lenses.

C) The receive Botox injections.

D) They are claustrophobic.

QUESTION 26:

Marisol meets a prospective client who wants eyelash extensions. The client wants to know whether they can safely receive lash extensions. They have chronic dry eyes, and they take prescription eye drops. What is Marisol most likely to tell the client?

A) Regular use of eye drops will compromise lash extensions.

B) People with dry eyes can get lash extensions just like anyone else.

C) They can get extensions if they switch to a specially formulated eye drop.

D) They can get classic extensions but not volume extensions.

QUESTION 27:

One of Marisol's clients is undergoing chemotherapy and has lost most of their eyelashes. Which of the following services can Marisol most likely provide to the client?

A) Apply mink lash extensions that are very light.

B) Apply volume lash extensions to make the lashes look thick.

C) Show them how to create a lash line using eyeliner.

D) Show them how to apply temporary lashes.

Ch. 06: Eyelash Extension Application

QUESTION 28:

Jishnu, a lash technician, has a prospective client who wants to know how big the treatment room is as they are a bit claustrophobic. Jishnu shows the room to the client, and the client approves the room and books an appointment for consultation. After the client leaves, Jishnu mentions to Marisol that their client has mild claustrophobia. What is Marisol likely to tell Jishnu to clearly communicate to the client?

A) They will have to keep their eyes closed for the entire duration of the service.

B) Claustrophobia contraindicates lash extension services.

C) The service cannot be stopped in between if they become uncomfortable during the service.

D) They must ask for breaks to open their eyes during the service whenever they find it difficult to keep their eyes closed.

QUESTION 29:

Yelda, a colleague of Marisol, has a client who wears glasses regularly. Yelda, who has never applied lash extensions to a person who wears glasses, asks for Marisol's advice. Which of the following is Marisol most likely to tell Yelda?

A) Apply the lashes as you would apply them for anyone.

B) Customize the lashes so that they do not touch the client's glasses when they blink.

C) Use J curl extensions to keep the look natural as that looks the best with glasses.

D) Keep the longest lashes toward the outer corner of the eyes.

Preparation for Extensions

 Learning Objective 06

Discuss how to prepare the client for lash application.

 Caution!

The client should keep their eyes closed during the entire procedure, and at no time should adhesive be allowed to enter the eye. If adhesive gets in the client's eye, follow emergency eye cleansing protocol: Flush with sterile eyewash solution and assist the client in washing their eyes with warm water for at least 15 minutes. Then, seek medical attention immediately.

Eyelash extension application happens close to the eye, so safety should be the number one priority. Follow all sterilization and disinfection guidelines for your equipment. In addition, incorporate as many single-use disposable products as possible. Wash your hands thoroughly before beginning the procedure.

Provide a comfortable place for your client to recline, ensuring the neck and head are adequately supported. This procedure can last up to several hours, and you want your client to be as comfortable as possible during that time.

- Ask the client to remove contact lenses before the procedure.
- Make sure you have a good light source, as this is important for proper application.
- Make sure saline or water is available close to your workstation in case you need to irrigate the eye for any reason.
- Clean and disinfect all tools before the procedure to ensure that you will not introduce bacteria into the client's eyes. Put on fresh nitrile gloves if you have not already.
- Handle tweezers only by the handle, never the tip, and always have an extra pair of tweezers available so you can disinfect one pair while you use the other pair on your next client.
- When removing lashes from their containers, use clean tweezers rather than your fingers.
- Dispose of all leftover lash extensions. Never put potentially contaminated lashes back into the container with new ones.

Taping Technique

Eye pads should be placed over the lower lashes, but not covering the entirety of the lashes. The job of the eye pads is to protect the skin from the tweezers while isolating, as well as to keep the lower lashes separated from the upper lashes. Keep in mind that placing the eye pads too close to the water line will result in bruising or cutting of the eye. This can be very painful for the client.

The surface of the eye pad is made with a very fine-fibered fabric. The fibers on the eye pad closest to the eye may become loose during the procedure, causing the upper lashes to stick to the fibers. Covering the upper edge of the pad with surgical tape will prevent this from being an issue. Use two strips of tape for each eye and apply the strips by crossing them at the center of the lash line at a slight angle to cover any exposed lower lashes **(Figure 6–5)**.

An alternative option is to place the tape directly on the lower lashes and the skin, making an eye pad unnecessary. If you are not careful, removing the tape from the skin can cause skin irritation or even tearing, so this method is not optimal.

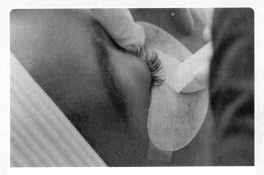

Fig. 6-5: Use tape to cover any exposed lower lashes.

 Here's a Tip

Colored eye pads and tape can be very helpful when working with blonde or light-colored lashes. If the client doesn't want to tint their lashes prior, colored tape will aid in your being able to see the natural lashes regardless of color.

Ch. 06: Eyelash Extension Application

Practice

Practicing any new technique is important. While you may be able to gain experience working on real clients in a school's student salon, another option is available to you. To practice, you will need a mannequin head and eyelash extension supplies. There are different types of mannequins. Some mannequins have removable eyelids with eyelashes, whereas others need a set of special strip training eyelashes to act as the client's upper natural lash **(Figure 6–6)**.

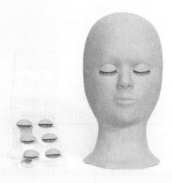

Fig. 6-6: Eyelash extension mannequin.

Here's a Tip

Create good habits by always placing a headband and under eye pads on your mannequin in preparation for lash extension services!

Check In

9. What is the purpose of eye pads?

Workbook Assessment

Fill in the blanks below using words from the provided word bank.

Fill in the Blank

QUESTION 30:

During an eyelash service, the client's eyes must remain .... at all times.

QUESTION 31:

Before starting a lash service, you must ensure that either .... or water is close by in case you have to irrigate the client's eye.

QUESTION 32:

In an eyelash procedure, before handling tweezers, the eyelash technician must wear .... gloves.

Word Bank

upper
handle
closed
tape
skin
fabric
lower
tip
saline
nitrile
tweezers
water line

Ch. 06: Eyelash Extension Application

QUESTION 33:

A lash technician must always hold a tweezer by its .... and never by its

....

QUESTION 34:

A lash technician must always use their .... to remove lash extensions from their container.

QUESTION 35:

Denali is preparing a client for eyelash extension application. They must place the gel eye pad on the client such that the eye pad covers the .... lashes. Denali must be careful to not place the eye pad too close to the .... as that can lead to injury to the eyes.

QUESTION 36:

The main purpose of the gel eye pad is to protect the .... from the

....

QUESTION 37:

The eye pad material is a(n) .... made of fine fibers. It can fray, and its fibers can hurt the eye. The lash technician can prevent the eye pad fabric from becoming loose by adhering two pieces of surgical

.... to the .... edge of the eye pad.

Ch. 06: Eyelash Extension Application

Temporary Eyelash Application

> **Learning Objective 07**
>
> Apply temporary cluster or strip lashes to the client safely.

Temporary lashes primarily differ from lash extensions by being faster to apply, being less expensive, and lasting a *much* shorter amount of time. Temporary lashes are usually used to add a dramatic flair for a single special event. They should be removed at the end of the day or event. During the consultation, discuss with your client their desired lash needs and whether temporary lashes or lash extensions are the better solution.

> **Caution!**
>
> Adhesive for temporary lashes is very different from adhesive for eyelash extensions! Make sure you are using the correct adhesive and understand its safety guidelines.

Types of Temporary Lashes

Three types of temporary artificial eyelashes are commonly used: strip, cluster, and individual lashes.

- Temporary **strip lashes**, also known as *band lashes*, are eyelash hairs on a strip applied with adhesive to the natural lash line. They cover the entire length of the lash line. If the eyelash band is too long to fit the curve of the upper eyelid, trim the outside edge. Before applying the lashes, use your fingers to bend the lash into a horseshoe shape so that it fits the contour of the eyelid. Temporary strip lashes come in a variety of colors and designs **(Figure 6–7)**.

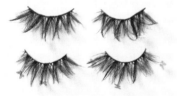

Fig. 6-7: Fashion strip lashes.

- **Individual lashes** are separate artificial eyelashes applied one at a time on top of the client's lashes. Individual lashes create a full, natural-looking lash line. Note that individual lashes are not the same as synthetic eyelash extensions that last 6 to 8 weeks.

- **Cluster lashes** are multiple artificial eyelashes grouped together at a short band or knotted base. They provide volume, length, and thickness in targeted sections instead of across the whole lash line like a strip lash. Cluster lashes are also referred to as tabs and are applied in a similar manner to individual temporary lashes.

> **Caution!**
>
> Temporary eyelash clusters should *never* be used as eyelash extensions. They attach to more than one lash and can cause damage to the natural lashes if left on for a long period of time.

> **Perform:**
>
> Perform 6-1: Temporary Eyelash Strip Application
>
> Perform 6-2: Temporary Eyelash Cluster Application

> **Here's a Tip**
>
> Never attempt to feather lash tips by nipping them with the points of your scissors. This results in blunt tips that look unnatural.

Removing Temporary Eyelashes

To remove artificial eyelashes, use eye pads saturated with an oil-based eye makeup remover formulated to remove waterproof mascara. The lash base may also be softened by applying a facecloth or cotton pad saturated with warm water and a gentle facial cleanser.

- Hold the cloth over the eyes for a few seconds to soften the adhesive.
- Starting from the outer corner, remove the lashes carefully to avoid pulling out the client's own lashes. If needed, apply facial cleanser with a cotton swab to dissolve adhesive.
- Pull strip lashes off parallel to the skin, not straight out.
- Use wet cotton pads or swabs to remove any makeup and adhesive remaining on the eyelid.

 Check In

10. Of the three types of temporary lashes, which can quickly add volume to the outside corner of the eye?

   ....
   ....
   ....

Workbook Assessment

Matching

For the following questions, match each statement to the correct letter choice.

QUESTION 38:

Match the types of temporary eyelashes with their descriptions.

............) The eyelash hairs in these lashes are situated on a band, which is glued to the natural lash line with an adhesive.

............) These are separate eyelash hairs that are applied one at a time on top of natural lash hairs.

............) These are a group of artificial lash hairs attached together to a short band.

Choices

A. cluster lashes
B. strip lashes
C. individual lashes

QUESTION 39:

Match the types of temporary lashes with their purpose.

............) These temporary eyelashes can be applied to the entire length of the natural lash line in a single piece.

............) These temporary lashes are used to create a full and natural-looking lash line. They also last longer than band lashes.

............) These temporary lashes are used to create volume, length, and thickness in targeted sections of the lash line.

Choices

A. individual lashes
B. cluster lashes
C. strip lashes

Classic Eyelash Application

 Learning Objective 08

Perform a classic eyelash application.

Classic eyelash applications are the most natural lash extension style you can offer. This is a great starting point for a lot of clients who are new to the lash world, as you can build many looks from a classic baseline. Classic extensions are utilized on a one-to-one basis, meaning that one single extension is applied to one single natural lash. Classic lashes are perfect for anyone wanting a more natural look but still wanting some lash enhancement. As always, the length, curl, and diameter are dependent upon the health, integrity, curl, length, and diameter of the natural lashes.

It is of the utmost importance to isolate the natural lash appropriately, place the lash extension correctly, use the appropriate amount of adhesive, and wait for the adhesive to dry before moving to the next lash. Although proper isolation certainly leads to better looking lashes, it also avoids *stickies*, extensions clumping together, which can put too much weight on the natural lashes. These clumps can cause damage to hair follicles and may lead to natural lash loss, not to mention discomfort and poor retention in the short term. There is little room for error in doing lash extensions, and attention to detail must be paid to avoid any discomfort or injury to the client. Proper isolation involves using your tweezers to separate natural lashes so that you can select the one single natural lash to attach the lash extension **(Figure 6-8)**. Follow the steps for classic eyelash application in **Procedure 6-3: Classic Eyelash Application.**

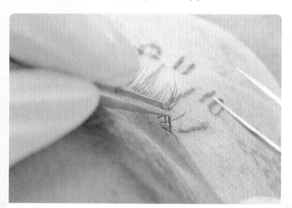

Fig. 6-8: Natural lash isolation.

 Perform:

Perform 6-3: Classic Eyelash Application

Lash Extension Placement

Extension placement on the natural lash looks, feels, and lasts better when done correctly. Consider these guidelines when placing lashes:

- Attach lashes no less than 1 mm and no more than 2 mm out from the lash line. Too close can cause discomfort from the glue or from the extension touching the eyelid skin. Too far leaves a visible space that can accumulate debris and can lead to the lash falling off.
- Ensure at least 2 mm of the natural lash and the lash extension are attached by following the curve of the natural lash. This will support the extension and avoid creating a space for dirt/debris to build up and push the lash off.
- Extensions should be applied at a 90-degree angle to the lash line.

Application Variation

It is recommended that you alternate back and forth between the eyes to keep them even and symmetrical. This method allows more drying time for adjacent lashes and a more balanced look if you run short on time and are unable to complete the process.

Another method involves applying lashes to one eye at a time. To do this, start with the centermost lash. Then, move to the outermost lash, then halfway between these two, and then halfway between the center lash and the inner corner of the eye. Once these are in place, go back to the center and start adding an adjacent lash next to each of the existing ones, rotating across the eye. Repeat this step until you have applied all the lashes. Then, move to the other eye and repeat the process.

Check In

11. Why is alternating between eyes during application less risky than completing one eye at a time?

....

....

....

Workbook Assessment

Fill in the Blank

Fill in the blanks below using words from the provided word bank.

QUESTION 40:

In a(n) .... eyelash application, each eyelash extension is applied to an individual natural lash.

QUESTION 41:

.... eyelash application is ideal for a person who wants to enhance their eyelashes but at the same time wants a natural look.

QUESTION 42:

When performing a classic eyelash application, you must place the eyelash extensions at least .... mm, and at the most .... mm, from the lash line.

QUESTION 43:

When performing a classic eyelash application, at least .... mm of the lash extension and the natural lash must be glued together. To avoid creating a space for debris between the extension and the natural lash, the extension must follow the

.... of the natural lash.

Word Bank

eyelid
tweezers
straight pointed tip
classic
centermost
dental mirror
downward
straight pointed tip
curved
isolation
micro swabs
inner
lash line
upper
outermost
1
nose
curve
2

Ch. 06: Eyelash Extension Application

QUESTION 44:

When performing a classic eyelash application, the angle between the .... and the lash extension should be 90 degrees unless otherwise specified in the lash map. If this angle is more than 90 degrees at the inner corner of the eye, the extensions may hit the client's ....

QUESTION 45:

To apply classic eyelash extensions to a client one eye at a time, you must first apply the extension to the .... lash, then to the .... lash, then to the lash that is in the center of the two, and then to the lash that is halfway between the centermost lash and the .... corner of the eye. You must then repeat the sequence by applying extensions to the lashes adjacent to the existing extensions until the application is complete.

QUESTION 46:

Proper .... of the lashes can help a lash technician avoid the clumping of extensions while applying classic eyelash extensions. The lash technician must use their .... to separate natural lashes and attached individual extensions to individual natural lash.

QUESTION 47:

During a classic eyelash application, if you are using a primer, you must apply it using two .... You must apply the primer to the top and the bottom of the .... lashes with a sweeping motion in a(n) .... direction.

QUESTION 48:

After completing a classic eyelash application, Uma wants to check for lashes stuck to the eye pad. To do so, Uma must pull back the client's .... with the nondominant hand and use .... tweezers with the dominant hand to separate stuck eyelashes from the eye pad.

Word Bank

eyelid
tweezers
straight pointed tip
classic
centermost
dental mirror
downward
straight pointed tip
curved
isolation
micro swabs
inner
lash line
upper
outermost
1
nose
curve
2

QUESTION 49:

After completing a classic eyelash application, a lash technician may use a(n) .... to check for lashes stuck to the lower lashes. To separate any stuck lashes, the technician must use .... tweezers to grasp the extension and the .... tweezers to grasp the lower natural lash and gently peel them apart.

Volume Eyelash Application

 Learning Objective 09

Perform a volume eyelash application.

Volume eyelash applications are some of the most tedious and difficult techniques you will learn. Volume techniques take a lot of skill, practice, dedication, and most of all, patience. Advanced skills include, but are not limited to, mega-volume, Russian volume, and wispy volume/strip lash style. These styles require the creation and use of **lash fans**, multiple single lash extensions in a group with a single base and fanned out at the tips.

- Mega volume is a very dramatic, dark set of lashes. If the natural lash can handle it, these fans can be made with up to 20 lashes in each fan.
- Russian volume is a difficult technique, focused on symmetry and precision.
- Strip lash or wispy style is asymmetrical and mimics the look of a strip lash. These sets do not look uniform, which is the selling point of that style.

 Here's a Tip

Keep in mind that you should not be aspiring to be good at every single one of these styles! Master the one you like the best and market yourself as an expert at it.

You can also purchase premade lash fans, which will help with your timing, but keep in mind that there is little customization with a premade fan.

Perfect lash fans are symmetrical with a 2 to 3 mm base, about one-third of the length of the fan, for adhesive **(Figure 6-9)**. The equal distance between single lashes is both appealing in its symmetry and leads to a nicer looking set that continues to look good as it wears.

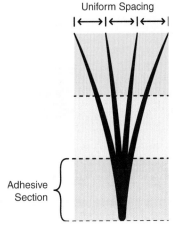

Fig. 6-9: The perfect lash fan.

Lash fans can be customized to create different looks.
- Narrow fans will create a full, thick look.
- Wide fans will create a feathery, not-as-bold look.
- Thin, pointed bases can be attached to the top or sides of natural lashes.
- Flat bases cannot be placed on the sides of the natural lash, but they can make the lash line look fuller.

Ch. 06: Eyelash Extension Application

Did You Know?

Lash fan volume numbers are determined by how many individual lashes are in the fan. 2D has two lash extensions, 3D has three lashes, 4D has four lashes, and so on! Remember that more weight is added with each additional extension. Always keep in mind what your client's natural lashes can handle!

Creating a Lash Fan

There are multiple techniques to create a lash fan. One of these techniques is not better than the other, so choose the technique that works best for you. Remember that they all take practice!

- Use the lash strip tape. You can pull the group of lashes and move them down the strip or leave them where they are. Either way, use your tweezers to gently fan the group of lashes out by applying pressure and twisting slightly **(Figure 6-10)**.

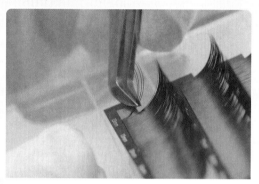

Fig. 6-10: Create a lash fan using the lash strip tape.

- Pinch the base and lightly twist into the desired shape using your gloved thumb and pointer finger.
- Use a sticky dot or square to place the fan and shape the fan using your tweezers.

Follow the steps for volume eyelash application in **Procedure 6-4: Volume Eyelash Application.** As with classic eyelash application, lash isolation, lash placement, and using the correct amount of adhesive are all extremely important to the success of the procedure and preventing any discomfort or injury to the client.

Perform:

Perform 6-4: Volume Eyelash Application

Check In

12. How much space should be at the base of a perfect lash fan for adhesive?

    ....

    ....

    ....

Workbook Assessment

For the following questions, match each statement to the correct letter choice.

Matching

QUESTION 50:

Match the types of volume lash techniques with their descriptions.

............) a very dramatic, dark set of lashes

............) a very symmetric and precise set of lashes

............) an asymmetrical set of lashes that does not look uniform

Choices
A. Russian volume lashes
B. strip lash
C. mega volume lashes

QUESTION 51:

Match the type of lash fans with the looks that can be created with them.

............) a full, thick look

............) a feathery, not too bold look

............) can be placed to the tops, sides, or bottom of natural lashes

............) make the lash line look fuller but cannot be placed on the sides of the natural lashes

Choices
A. wide lash fans
B. lash fans with thin, pointed bases
C. lash fans with flat bases
D. narrow lash fans

Eyelash Refill

 Learning Objective 10

Perform an eyelash refill procedure.

An **eyelash refill** is a procedure in which the outgrown lash extensions are removed, new lashes are put in their place, and new lash extensions are added to natural lashes that have moved from the anagen phase to the catagen phase of growth. Also called *lash fills*, they are recommended every 2 to 3 weeks. Three weeks is the maximum amount of time that extensions can safely be worn. Keeping outgrown lashes on can result in follicle damage or painful twisting lashes. During the refill service, any lash extensions that have grown out by 1 mm or more from their original placement should be removed (**Figure 6-11**). Once these outgrown lashes are removed, proceed with applying lash extensions in those spaces. Moving back and forth between the two eyes, proceed until every lash is completed. Follow the steps for eyelash refill in **Procedure 6-5: Eyelash Refill**.

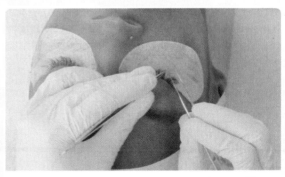

Fig. 6-11: Remove outgrown lashes during a refill service first.

Ch. 06: Eyelash Extension Application

Educating your clients on why refills are necessary is very important. Lash extensions are a commitment and an investment, with maintenance required to maintain the look of the lashes. Notify your client that 40 percent of their lash extensions must remain to consider their appointment a refill. Showing up with anything less than 40 percent will result in a full removal and a new full set. You may need to reschedule to another day to account for proper service time.

Perform:

Perform 6-5: Eyelash Refill

Focus On

Service Timing

Lash extensions take a significant amount of time. When you're in school, full sets can range from four to six hours, and fills can be two hours. As you get more comfortable with your skills, you *will* be able to cut down the length of time that is booked; however, doing something quickly does not mean you are doing it correctly. As you are learning, focus on performing the service correctly and over time you will begin to do it more quickly. Do not worry about your timing; worry about the precision and skill set you are embodying.

Check In

13. How often should a client come in for lash refills?

   ....

   ....

   ....

Workbook Assessment

Please circle the correct answer for each question below.

Multiple Choice

QUESTION 52:

Your client's eyelash extensions look a bit unkempt as some of them appear overgrown. The client wants you to remove the outgrown lashes and apply new extensions in their place. In the given scenario, what does the client need?

   A) eyelash refill service

   B) volume eyelash application

   C) cluster lash application

   D) band lash service

QUESTION 53:

What is the maximum duration for which eyelash extensions can be safely worn without getting an eyelash refill?

   A) 5 weeks

   B) 1 week

   C) 3 weeks

   D) 8 weeks

QUESTION 54:

Which of the following should you do while performing an eyelash refill service for a client?

A) Reattach extensions that are peeling away from the natural lash.

B) Apply adhesive remover to remove all the lash extensions.

C) Trim extensions that have outgrown the natural lash.

D) Remove extensions that have moved 1 mm or more from their original position.

QUESTION 55:

Which of the following would you do if the peeling method of lash removal does not work on an outgrown lash extension?

A) Use an adhesive remover.

B) Cut the extension close to the point of attachment to the natural lash.

C) Leave the lash as it is.

D) Pluck out the natural lash to which the extension is attached.

QUESTION 56:

For a lash service to be considered an eyelash refill, what is the lowest percentage of intact lashes? If the percentage of intact lashes is less than that, it is considered a full service.

A) 10%

B) 40%

C) 60%

D) 20%

Eyelash Extension Removal

Learning Objective 11

Perform an eyelash extension removal service.

When removing lash extensions, great caution should be followed when using a chemical remover. Clients should lie down at an incline or sit upright to prevent adhesive from entering their eyes. Chemical removers come in liquid, cream, or gel form **(Figure 6-12)**. Chemical removers are very potent and dissolve the bond of the lash adhesive from the natural lash. This solution should only be used on closed eyes, with saline or water available in case of an emergency. Follow the steps for eyelash extension removal in **Procedure 6-6: Eyelash Extension Removal.**

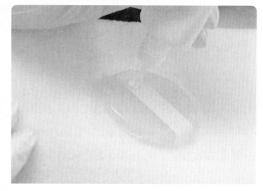

Fig. 6-12: Gel chemical remover.

 Perform:

Perform 6-6: Eyelash Extension Removal

Manual removal can be performed on lash extensions that do not have an excess amount of adhesive on them. Simply use the *banana peel method*, which begins by holding the natural lash with the tips of one tweezer. With the other tweezer, gently peel the extension away from the natural lash, removing it from the bond. Keep in mind that this technique will only be successful on lashes that are applied properly, with the appropriate amount of adhesive.

If during the removal process you cannot remove certain extensions, wipe the client's eyes with damp cotton rounds to cleanse adhesive remover, replace the eye pads, and manually remove stubborn lashes with your tweezers. Wipe several times thoroughly, ensuring the remover is completely gone prior to the client opening their eyes.

 Caution!

Never use dry cotton on or near lash extensions. The reaction of the lash adhesive and cotton causes heat and can burn the client or technician.

 Check In

14. Why does the client need to lie on an incline during the chemical removal procedure?

Workbook Assessment

Fill in the blanks below using words from the provided word bank.

Fill in the Blank

QUESTION 57:

Belén's client wants to change their eyelash extensions from classic to volume eyelashes. To prepare the client for the eyelash removal, Belén must set the table

for the client at a(n) .... to prevent the adhesive or .... from getting into the client's eyes.

QUESTION 58:

Chemical .... work by dissolving the bond between the lash adhesive and the natural lash.

QUESTION 59:

Armondo is performing a lash removal service without using an adhesive remover.

They are using the .... method, in which they use tweezers to gently peel away the extensions from the natural lash. It a manual technique of lash extension

removal and whether it will work or not depends on the amount of ....

QUESTION 60:

When wiping the lash adhesive remover from a client's lashes, a lash technician must

never use .... as it reacts with the lash adhesive to produce heat, which can burn the client or the technician.

QUESTION 61:

Chemical adhesive removers are available in liquid, cream, and .... forms.

QUESTION 62:

While performing a lash removal service, after the adhesive remover has been

applied and processed, you must use two .... to stroke the lashes in a(n)

.... motion until all extensions come out.

Word Bank

outward
adhesive
lint-free applicators
straight
banana peel
adhesive removers
gel
adhesive remover
curved
incline
dry cotton

Ch. 06: Eyelash Extension Application

QUESTION 63:

For single lash removal, a lash technician must apply the .... to the lash and leave it on for 2 to 3 minutes. To remove the extension, the technician must use their dominant hand to hold the extension with a(n) .... tweezer and their nondominant hand to hold the natural lash with a(n) .... tweezer and gently pull the extension away from the natural lash.

Word Bank

outward
adhesive
lint-free applicators
straight
banana peel
adhesive removers
gel
adhesive remover
curved
incline
dry cotton

Client Aftercare

 Learning Objective 12

Describe aftercare instructions for eyelash extension clients.

Lash extensions will wear better and last longer if they are properly cared for at home. The following list provides general aftercare instructions for the client. Always be sure to follow the manufacturer's guidelines if they vary from this list, but these directives are a good starting point.

- Keep dry for 24 hours. Avoid water, makeup, skin care products, and so forth.
- Avoid hot steam or swimming for 48 hours.
- Avoid using any product on the bonded area of your new lashes and avoid using oil-based products of any kind near the eyes, especially oil-based eye makeup remover.
- Do not rub your eyes or pick at the lashes.
- Do not use mascara and avoid heavy eye makeup.
- Do not use mechanical eyelash curlers. These can damage lash extensions and break the bond of the adhesive.
- Wash the lashes with a lash cleanser, dry them, and brush them gently twice a day.
- Avoid sleeping on your lashes. Try sleeping on your back.
- Do not try to remove the extensions. Only allow a professional to remove them.

 Did You Know?

Correctly applied eyelashes will eliminate the need for mascara.

Show the client how to properly cleanse the lashes while the client is on your table. Pump lash cleanser onto a cleansing brush and sweep down onto the lashes in a downward motion. Rinse with water and brush the extensions.

Finally, ensure that the client has another appointment booked with you prior to them leaving your salon! This is also a fine time to offer some of the many aftercare retail options available—at least a cleanser and soft brush if they haven't been given one **(Figure 6–13)**. Refer to Chapter 8, Building an Eyelash Business, for more information.

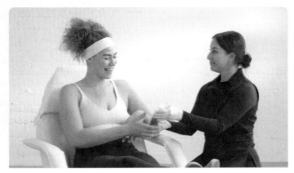

Fig. 6-13: Recommend lash cleanser at the end of a service.

 Here's a Tip

Creating aftercare cards with the tips above to hand out to clients is always helpful!

 Check In

15. Name three things a client should avoid after getting lash extensions.

....

....

....

Workbook Assessment

Select whether the statements below are true or false.

True or False

QUESTION 64:

Eyelash technicians must instruct their eyelash extension clients to wash their faces with only water for the first 24 hours after eyelash extension application.

T F why?..

QUESTION 65:

Clients must avoid hot steam or saunas for at least 48 hours after the application of eyelash extensions.

T F why?..

QUESTION 66:

Celio, a lash technician, gets a call from a client who has received eyelash extensions for the first time. The client says that while there is no real discomfort, the lashes feel odd and heavy. The client asks if there is something they can do to relieve the weird feeling. Celio must tell the client to use their index fingertip to gently rub the base of the lashes but avoid touching the lashes with the fingernail.

T F why?..

QUESTION 67:

Nuria, who has J curl eyelash extensions, wants to curl their extensions to create a dramatic look for a special occasion. The recommended way to achieve this look is to use mascara and a mechanical eyelash curler.

T F why?..

Ch. 06: Eyelash Extension Application

QUESTION 68:

If a person with eyelash extensions uses eye makeup, they must avoid makeup that requires oil-based makeup remover.

T F why?..

QUESTION 69:

After the lash extensions have been applied, a cleaning brush with lash cleanser must be swept down onto lashes in a downward motion.

T F why?..

Troubleshooting

 Learning Objective 13

Identify solutions to common eyelash extension problems.

As discussed, lash extensions are a very precise, technical skill set. Something so exacting comes with common issues most lash technicians will run into repeatedly in their careers. Consider the following situations and their solutions.

- **Too much adhesive is used.** It is important that the appropriate amount of adhesive is used during any lash appointment; however, if you use too much adhesive this doesn't mean the lash set is ruined! Instruct the client to remain still and keep their eyes closed. Use the banana peel method to remove the current extension, ensuring that the adhesive does not touch any other surrounding lashes. If the banana peel method is unsuccessful, place a small amount of lash remover onto the single lash, wait five minutes, and remove. If the neighboring lashes do get touched with the adhesive, repeat the step with the lash remover until the lashes are no longer clumped together.
- **Direction of the extension is incorrect.** Natural lashes can grow in different directions. That said, it is important to place extensions at a 90-degree angle from the lash line to ensure uniformity when the client opens their eyes. If you notice an extension is not placed correctly and the adhesive is still malleable, you can correct this by simply moving it into place and holding the isolation until the adhesive is dry. If the misplaced extension is noticed after the adhesive is dried, use the banana peel method to remove the extension and reapply. Keep in mind the dry time of the adhesive you are using. Most lash adhesives have a 0.5 to 2 second dry time, and movement of an extension cannot be done if the adhesive is dried.
- **Lash is getting stuck to the eye pad.** This is a very common occurrence and does not mean you are using too much adhesive. If this happens, gently lift the client's eyelid with your nondominant hand and use the tips of your tweezers in your dominant hand to unstick the extension from the eye pad. You may need to remove the extension if remnants of the eye pad are stuck to the extension.
- **Client's eyes are watering.** This is another common occurrence that can be caused by fumes, bright light, eye pads, or from them talking or laughing. Use a lint free adhesive wipe to soak up any moisture surrounding the eyes—remember that cotton products should never be used near lash extensions. If there is too much moisture, replacing the eye pads may be necessary. To do this, dry the lashes thoroughly and remove the tape and eye pads. Ask the client to blot their eyes. Then, replace the pads and tape as usual.
- **Lash extensions fall off too early.** Lash retention is a very popular topic, with several factors coming into play. If a client is experiencing excessive premature lash extension loss, check in with them regarding the following:
    - Did they wait 24 hours before wetting the lashes?
    - Are they wearing waterproof (oily) makeup?
    - Are they picking and pulling at the lashes?
    - Are they properly cleansing the lashes daily with an appropriate cleanser?
    - Do they have a condition or medication that was not disclosed on the consent form?

You should also circle back and check in with yourself:

- Is my adhesive fresh, properly stored, and of good quality?
- Did I use enough adhesive?
- Did I clean their lashes properly?
- Did I apply extensions on lashes too far in their growth cycle?
- Did I give the appropriate aftercare guidelines?

Lash retention is a 50/50 relationship! Educate clients on proper aftercare and be transparent about the realities of premature lash extension loss if aftercare is not followed. If this is a consistent issue with a specific client, there is likely something they are doing at home that is affecting retention. Go over a list of what they are using at home and give product recommendations if necessary.

- **Natural lashes are damaged.** If you are doing lash extensions appropriately (correct weight, length, adhesive usage, etc.), there is no reason your client's natural lashes should be damaged. Damage comes from faulty application and product usage. Clients who pick at their lashes may also experience damage and potentially permanent lash loss in the areas picked off. If you notice damage, take photos and communicate with your client what you are noticing. Ask if they are picking and explain the damage that can be caused. When lashes are applied appropriately, the natural lashes should be able to grow and thrive.

✓ Check In

16. What should you do if the client's lashes get stuck to the eye pad?

17. Who is ultimately responsible for lash retention?

Workbook Assessment

Multiple Choice

Please circle the correct answer for each question.

Zarina is a trainee lash technician who must practice at least 12 full services before they can start charging full price for applying lash extension. Zarina's friend Mala agrees to let them practice on her eyelashes.

QUESTION 70:

While applying lashes to Mala, Zarina notices that some of the lashes have clumped together. Zarina is not sure of the cause of the clumping and asks her supervisor, Eduardo, for his advice. Which of the following is Eduardo most likely to tell Zarina?

A) Zarina is using too much adhesive.

B) Zarina is not placing the lashes at a 90-degree angle to the lash line.

C) The client's eyes are watering.

D) The adhesive is curing too quickly.

QUESTION 71:

After applying few lashes, Zarina notices that some of the eyelashes are stuck to the gel eye pad. Which of the following should Zarina use to separate the lashes from the eye pad?

A) an adhesive remover

B) water

C) tweezers

D) a lash cleanser

QUESTION 72:

A few minutes into the service, Mala complains of slight discomfort in one of the eyes. Zarina notices a slight bruising in the eye. Which of the following could be a likely reason for this?

A) The lash adhesive is drying too quickly.

B) Mala has fallen asleep during the lash application process.

C) The fumes from the lash adhesive are causing an allergic reaction.

D) Zarina has placed the eye pad too close to Mala's water line.

QUESTION 73:

After correcting the position of the eye pad, Mala's eye no longer hurts, and she is comfortable to continue with the extension application. After about half an hour, Mala's eyes become slightly watery because of the fumes of the adhesive. What should Zarina do?

A) Use a lint free adhesive wipe to absorb the moisture around the eyes.

B) Ignore the watering as it is minimal.

C) Stop the service and reschedule the appointment.

D) Place a piece of cotton at the corner of the eye to soak up any moisture.

QUESTION 74:

A few days after the lash extension application, Mala returns to the salon and tells Zarina that her lash extensions are falling off. Zarina asks Mala a few questions to ascertain the reason for poor lash retention. Which of the following is most likely the reason why Mala's lashes have poor retention?

A) Mala has been brushing the lashes twice a day.

B) Mala has been using waterproof eye makeup.

C) Mala has been sleeping on her back.

D) Mala went swimming 3 days after lash application.

Chapter Glossary

classic eyelash application *KLA-suhk AI-lash a-pluh-KAY-shun*	p. 132	service in which single eyelash extensions are applied to single natural eyelashes
cluster lashes *KLUH-stur LA-shuhz*	p. 130	multiple artificial eyelashes grouped together at a short band or knotted base
contraindications *kahn-TRAH-in-dih-KAY-shuns*	p. 124	situations in which eyelash extensions should not be applied because they could cause harm to the client
eyelash refill *AI-lash REE-fil*	p. 137	procedure in which the outgrown eyelash extensions are removed and new eyelash extensions are put in their place
glaucoma *glaa-KOW-muh*	p. 124	disease in which the optic nerve is damaged and can lead to progressive, irreversible loss of vision
individual lashes *in-duh-VI-joo-uhl LA-shuhz*	p. 130	separate artificial eyelashes applied one at a time on top of the client's lashes
lash fans *lash fanz*	p. 135	multiple single eyelash extensions grouped together with a single base and fanned out tips
lash map *lash map*	p. 120	guide for placing specific lengths of lash extensions in a set
strip lashes *strip LA-shuhz*	p. 130	also known as *band lashes*; eyelash hairs on a strip applied with adhesive to the natural lash line
volume eyelash application *vol-YOOM AI-lash a-pluh-KAY-shun*	p. 135	service in which eyelash extensions are made into lash fans and applied to single natural eyelashes

Procedure 6-1: Temporary Eyelash Strip Application

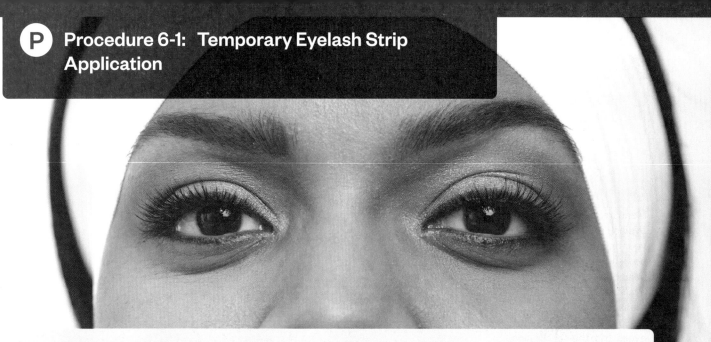

IMPLEMENTS AND MATERIALS:

- Adjustable LED light
- Artificial strip eyelashes
- Disposable mascara brushes
- Disposable micro swabs
- Disposable toothpick rounded (optional)
- Eyelash curler (optional)
- Eyeliner brush (optional)
- Gloves
- Jade stone or adhesive tray (sterilized and taped or disposable)
- Temporary eyelash adhesive
- Trimming scissors
- Slant tweezers

PREPARATION:

Perform Procedure 4-3: Pre-Service Procedure

PROCEDURE:

10 MIN

BEFORE

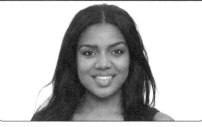

STEP 1

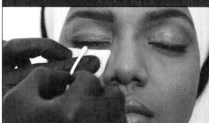

Brush the client's eyelashes. Ensure the lashes are clean and free of foreign matter, such as mascara particles. If needed, cleanse the client's eyelashes.

STEP 2

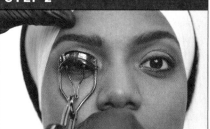

Curl the eyelashes with an eyelash curler (if desired). Curl before you apply the artificial lashes.

STEP 3

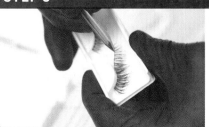

Carefully remove the eyelash band from the package using tweezers.

148   Ch. 06: Eyelash Extension Application

Procedure 6-1: Temporary Eyelash Strip Application

STEP 4

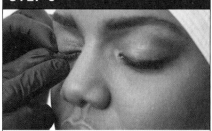

Measure the length of the upper eyelash and trim (if necessary). Use your fingers to bend the lash into a horseshoe shape to make it more flexible so it fits the contour of the eyelid. Hold the strip up to the eye to measure the length. If the band lash is too long to fit the curve of the upper eyelid, trim the outside edge.

Tip: You may wish to apply eyeliner before the lash is applied if it will not affect the false lash adhesion.

STEP 5

Apply a thin strip of lash adhesive to the base of the false lashes and allow it to set for a few seconds. Use a disposable micro swab or rounded end of a toothpick to apply the lash adhesive.

Note: Dispense lash adhesive onto a taped jade stone or disposable adhesive tray.

STEP 6

Apply the strip lashes. Apply the lashes by holding the ends with your fingers or tweezers. Start with the shorter part of the lash and place it on the inner corner of the lash line.

Tip: If applying individual temporary lashes, apply them one at a time, evenly spaced across the lash line. Use longer lashes on the outer edges of the eye, medium in the middle, and short on the inside corners.

STEP 7

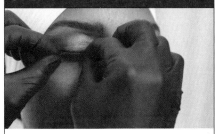

Position the rest of the lash as close to the client's natural lashes as possible. Remove any excess glue and reposition the lashes as necessary. Use tweezers or the rounded end of a lash liner brush to press the lash on without adhering the tweezers or brush to the glue.

Tip: Ask your client to keep their eyes slightly open to prevent the lashes from sticking to their lower lashes.

STEP 8

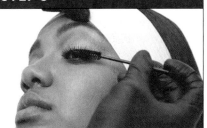

Apply liquid liner and mascara if desired. An additional liquid liner may be used to finish the look if it does not affect the false lash adhesion. Adding a coat of mascara can help false lashes adhere to natural lashes.

Optional: Apply the lower lash, if desired, following the same steps. Place the lash beneath the client's lower natural lash.

STEP 9

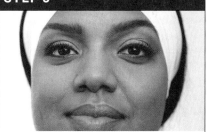

Show the client the finished look with a hand mirror and make sure the client is comfortable with the lashes.

Tip: Remind the client to take special care with artificial lashes when swimming, bathing, and cleansing the face. Water, oil, or cleansing products will loosen artificial lashes. Band lash applications last 1 day and are meant to be removed nightly.

POST SERVICE

Perform Procedure 4-4: Post-Service Procedure

Ch. 06: Eyelash Extension Application

Procedure 6-2: Temporary Eyelash Cluster Application

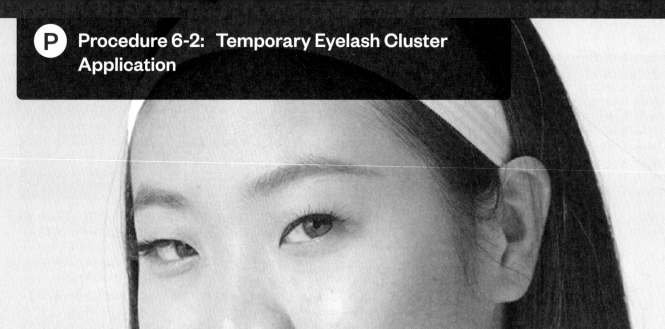

IMPLEMENTS AND MATERIALS:

- Adjustable LED light
- Artificial cluster eyelashes
- Disposable lint-free applicators
- Disposable mascara brushes
- Distilled water
- Eyelash cleanser
- Eyelash curler (optional)
- Eyeliner brush (optional)
- Gloves
- Jade stone
- Temporary eyelash adhesive
- Mini fan
- Paper towels
- Slant tweezers
- Squeeze bottle
- Surgical paper tape
- Trimming scissors

PREPARATION:

Perform Procedure 4-3: Pre-Service Procedure

PROCEDURE:

 20 MIN

BEFORE

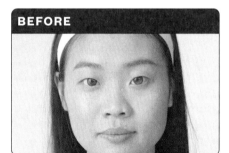

STEP 1

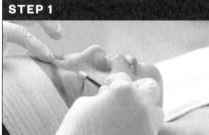

With the client lying down, sit behind them and cleanse the lashes in a downward motion using an eyelash cleanser and disposable lint-free applicators. Tilt the client's head to the side and, holding a folded paper towel to the side of their face, rinse with distilled water from a squeeze bottle.

Procedure 6-2: Temporary Eyelash Cluster Application

STEP 2

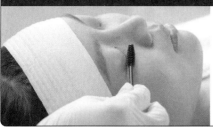

Gently pat the eye dry with the paper towel and repeat on the other eye. Thoroughly dry the lashes by brushing them through with a mascara brush and a mini fan. Ask the client to change to a seated position that is slightly reclined.

Note: If the client's lashes are straight, they can be curled with an eyelash curler before you apply the artificial lashes. You may wish to apply eyeliner before the lash is applied if it will not affect the false lash adhesion.

STEP 3

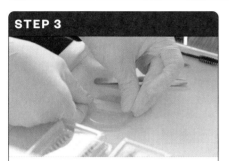

Cut and apply two overlapping strips of tape to the top of the jade stone.

STEP 4

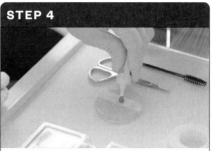

Place a small amount of adhesive on the jade stone or adhesive holder.

Caution: Make sure that you are using false eyelash adhesive and not lash extension adhesive.

STEP 5

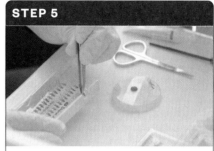

Placing yourself at the client's side, carefully remove the appropriately sized cluster lash from the package using tweezers.

STEP 6

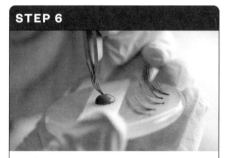

Dip the base of the lash cluster into the adhesive and allow a few seconds for the adhesive to set.

STEP 7

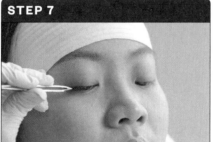

Apply one cluster at a time as close to the client's natural lashes as possible, working your way from the outer corner to the inner corner. Instruct your client to keep their eyes slightly open to prevent the cluster from sticking to the lower lashes.

STEP 8

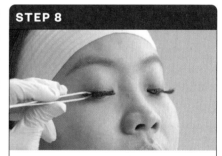

Using tweezers or the rounded end of an eyeliner brush, press the lash cluster on without touching the glue.

Optional: Apply the cluster lashes to the lower eyelashes. Ask your client to keep their eyes open while you place the clusters beneath the client's lower natural lashes.

Procedure 6-2: Temporary Eyelash Cluster Application

STEP 9

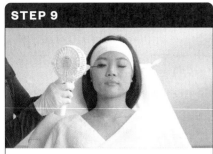

Once the lash clusters have been applied, use a mini fan to ensure the adhesive is dry.

STEP 10

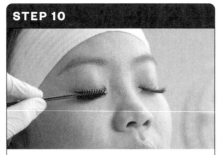

Gently brush the lashes with a mascara brush to blend the natural lashes with the clusters, avoiding contact with the base of the lash line.

STEP 11

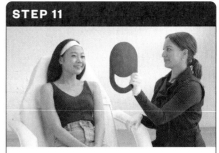

Show the client the finished look with a hand mirror and make sure the client is comfortable with the lashes.

POST SERVICE

Perform Procedure 4–4: Post-Service Procedure

Procedure 6-3: Classic Eyelash Application

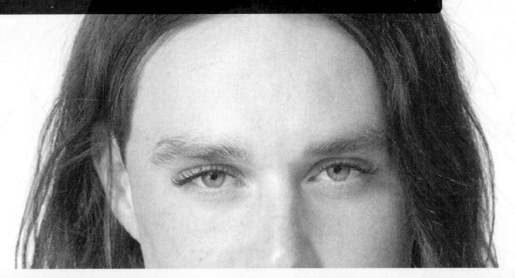

IMPLEMENTS AND MATERIALS:

- Adjustable LED light
- Assortment of individual eyelash extensions
- Dental mirror
- Disposable lint-free applicators
- Disposable mascara brushes
- Disposable micro swabs
- Distilled water
- Eyelash cleanser
- Eyelash extension adhesive
- Fine felt-tipped marker
- Gloves
- Jade stone or adhesive holder
- Lash primer (optional)
- Lash tile or palette
- Longer life coating sealant (optional)
- Mini fan
- Paper towels
- Squeeze bottle
- Surgical paper tape
- Trimming scissors
- Tweezers, curved
- Tweezers, straight pointed tip
- Under-eye gel pads

PREPARATION:

Perform Procedure 4-3: Pre-Service Procedure

PROCEDURE:

 150 MIN

BEFORE	STEP 1	STEP 2
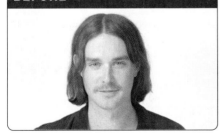	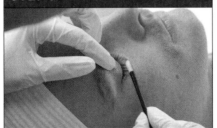	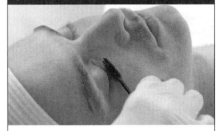
	With the client lying down, sit behind them and cleanse the lashes in a downward motion using an eyelash cleanser and disposable lint-free applicators. Tilt the client's head to the side and, holding a folded paper towel to the side of their face, rinse with distilled water from a squeeze bottle.	Gently pat the eye dry with the paper towel and repeat on the other eye. Thoroughly dry the lashes by brushing them through with a mascara brush and a mini fan. *Tip: If needed, repeat the cleansing process again until the eyelashes are free of residue.*

Ch. 06: Eyelash Extension Application

Procedure 6-3: Classic Eyelash Application

STEP 3

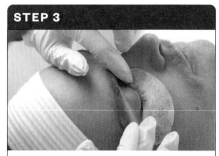

Remove the gel pads from their protective backing. While gently pulling back the client's eyelid, position the gel pads under each eye by covering the lower lash line. Be careful not to touch the inner eye rim.

STEP 4

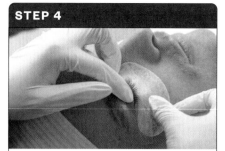

Cut two strips of surgical tape for each eye. Apply the strips under each eye by crossing them at the center of the lash line at a slight angle to cover any exposed lower lashes.

Tip: Always check in with your client to make sure the tape and pads are comfortable.

STEP 5

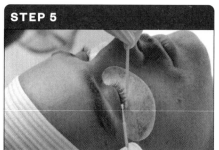

If you are using eyelash primer, apply a small amount to two micro swabs and apply to the bottom and top of the upper lashes using a downward sweeping motion. Dry with a mini fan.

STEP 6

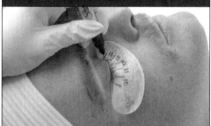

Map the lash pattern guide from your style consultation onto the gel pads with a fine felt-tipped marker. Choose the lashes according to the lash map and, using tweezers, place them onto the lash tile or palette.

STEP 7

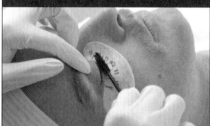

Gently comb through the client's natural lashes with a mascara brush to straighten them.

STEP 8

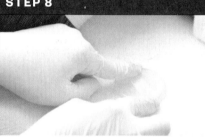

Cut two strips of surgical tape. Apply the strips by overlapping them on top of the jade stone or tile.

STEP 9

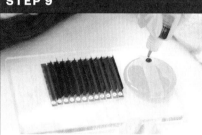

Shake the adhesive well and place a pea-sized drop on to the taped jade stone, the tile, or a disposable adhesive holder.

Tip: Remember to replace the adhesive with a fresh dot every 15 to 20 minutes.

STEP 10

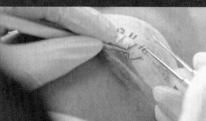

Starting at the outside corner of the eye, isolate a single natural lash using the curved tweezers in your nondominant hand.

STEP 11

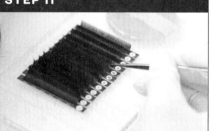

With straight pointed-tip tweezers in your dominant hand, pick up an eyelash extension by the tapered end.

Procedure 6-3: Classic Eyelash Application

STEP 12

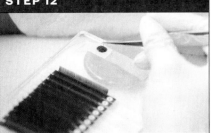

Slowly dip 1/4 of the thick end of the eyelash extension into the center of the adhesive dot. If you see droplets on the extension, re-dip into the center of the adhesive drop to remove excess adhesive.

Caution!
Do not swipe excess adhesive off, as it begins the curing process and can compromise your adhesion.

STEP 13

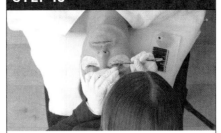

Place the extension on top of the isolated eyelash roughly 1 to 2 mm from the base of the lash line, avoiding contact with the skin. Guide the extension to match the angle of your client's natural lash curve.

STEP 14

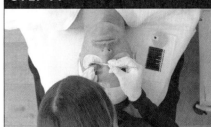

Repeat Steps 10 through 13 on the opposite eye, alternating between each eye to ensure proper drying time. Place the lashes at spaced intervals to avoid sticking or clumping.

STEP 15

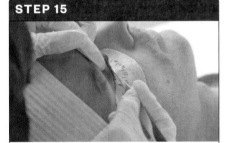

Check for lashes sticking to the eye pads by gently pulling back your client's eyelid with your nondominant hand and, using the straight pointed-tip tweezers in your dominant hand, gently unstick lashes from the eye pads if needed.

Tip: You should check for sticking several times during the procedure.

STEP 16

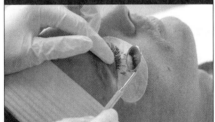

Check for lashes sticking to any lower lashes by using a dental mirror while gently pulling back your client's eyelid. If the client's eyelashes are stuck together, grasp the extension with the curved tweezers in your nondominant hand, grasp the lower natural lash with the straight pointed-tip tweezers in your dominant hand, and gently peel them apart.

STEP 17

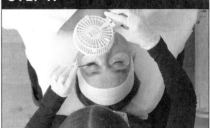

Once all eyelash extensions are in place, brush through them with a mascara brush and dry with a mini fan.

Note: If you are using a sealant or bonder, apply it with disposable micro swabs before drying the lashes.

STEP 18

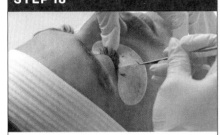

Remove the strips of tape first and then the eye pads to avoid pulling out any lower lashes that may be tucked between the pad and tape.

STEP 19

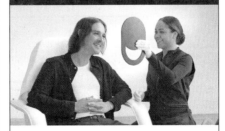

Show the client the finished look with a hand mirror and make sure the client is comfortable with the lashes.

POST SERVICE

Perform Procedure 4–4: Post-Service Procedure

Procedure 6-4: Volume Eyelash Application

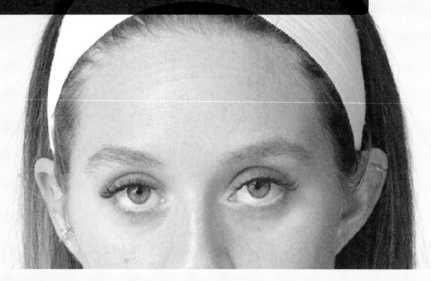

IMPLEMENTS AND MATERIALS:

- Adjustable LED light
- Assortment of individual eyelash extensions
- Dental mirror
- Disposable lint-free applicators
- Disposable mascara brushes
- Disposable micro swabs
- Distilled water
- Eyelash cleanser
- Eyelash extension adhesive
- Fine felt-tipped marker
- Gloves
- Jade stone or adhesive holder
- Lash primer (optional)
- Lash tile or palette
- Mini fan
- Paper towels
- Squeeze bottle
- Surgical paper tape
- Trimming scissors
- Tweezers, boot tip
- Tweezers, curved
- Under-eye gel pad

PREPARATION:

Perform Procedure 4-3: Pre-Service Procedure

PROCEDURE:

 210 MIN

BEFORE

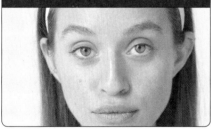

STEP 1

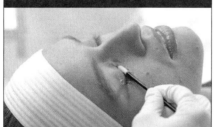

With the client lying down, sit behind them and cleanse the lashes in a downward motion using eyelash cleanser and disposable lint-free applicators. Tilt the client's head to the side and, holding a folded paper towel to the side of their face, rinse with distilled water from a squeeze bottle.

STEP 2

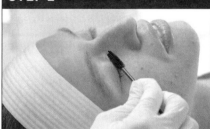

Gently pat the eye dry with the paper towel and repeat on the other eye. Thoroughly dry the lashes by brushing them through with a mascara brush and a mini fan.

Tip: If needed, repeat the cleansing process again until the eyelashes are free of residue.

Procedure 6-4: Volume Eyelash Application

STEP 3

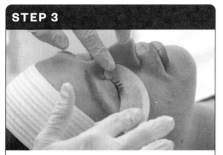

Remove the gel pads from their protective backing. While gently pulling back the client's eyelid, position the gel pads under each eye by covering the lower lash line. Be careful not to touch the inner eye rim.

STEP 4

Cut two strips of surgical tape for each eye. Apply the strips under each eye by crossing them at the center of the lash line at a slight angle to cover any exposed lower lashes.

Tip: Always check in with your client to make sure the tape and pads are comfortable.

STEP 5

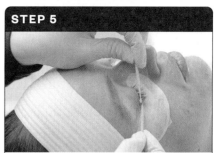

If you are using eyelash primer, apply a small amount to two micro swabs and apply it to the bottom and top of the upper lashes using a downward sweeping motion. Dry with a mini fan.

STEP 6

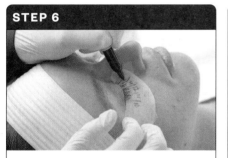

Map the lash pattern guide from your style consultation onto the gel pads with a fine felt-tipped marker. Choose the lashes according to the lash map and, using tweezers, place them onto the lash tile or palette.

STEP 7

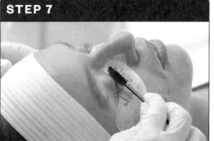

Gently comb through the client's natural lashes with a mascara brush to straighten them.

STEP 8

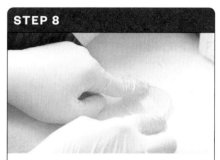

Cut two strips of surgical tape. Apply the strips by overlapping them on top of the jade stone or tile.

STEP 9

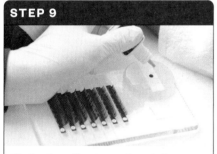

Shake the adhesive well and place a pea-sized drop onto the taped jade stone, the tile, or a disposable adhesive holder.

Tip: Remember to replace the adhesive with a fresh dot every 15 to 20 minutes.

STEP 10

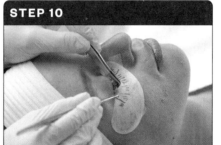

Starting at the outside corner of the eye, isolate a single natural lash using the curved tweezers in your nondominant hand.

STEP 11

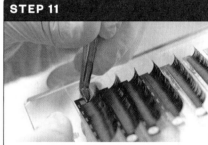

With boot tip tweezers in your dominant hand, grasp a group of eyelash extensions and gently pull toward you to separate them from the rest of the eyelash extensions. Create a lash fan by placing the extensions on the strip and using your tweezers to pick the fan open.

Tip: You can also create lash fans using other methods, such as the pinching technique.

Ch. 06: Eyelash Extension Application

Procedure 6-4: Volume Eyelash Application

STEP 12

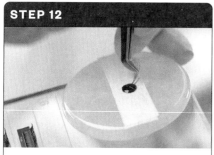

Grasp the lash fan in the sweet spot of the tweezers and slowly dip 0.5 mm of the base into the center of the adhesive dome, leaving a tiny drop of adhesive at the base of the lash fan. Too much adhesive will collapse the fan.

Caution!
Do not swipe excess adhesive off, as it begins the curing process and can compromise your adhesion.

STEP 13

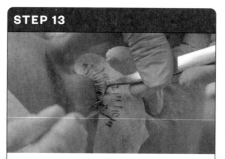

Place the lash fan on top of the isolated eyelash, roughly 1 to 2 mm from the base of the lash line, avoiding contact with the skin. The lash fan should wrap around the natural lash.

STEP 14

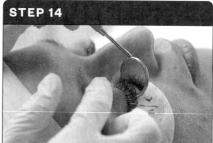

Repeat Steps 10 through 13 on the opposite eye, alternating between each eye to ensure proper drying time. Place the lashes at spaced intervals to avoid sticking or clumping and use your dental mirror to check for symmetry and any gaps.

STEP 15

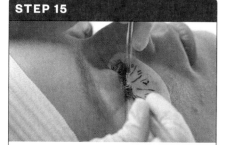

Check for lashes sticking to the eye pads by gently pulling back your client's eyelid with your nondominant hand and, using the boot tip tweezers in your dominant hand, gently unstick lashes from the eye pads if needed.

Tip: You should check for sticking several times during the procedure.

STEP 16

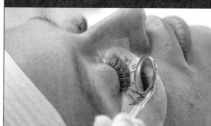

Check for lashes sticking to any lower lashes by using a dental mirror while gently pulling back your client's eyelid. If the client's eyelashes are stuck together, grasp the lash fan with the curved tweezers in your nondominant hand, grasp the lower natural lash with the boot tip tweezers in your dominant hand, and gently peel them apart.

STEP 17

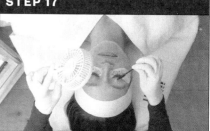

Once all eyelash extensions are in place, brush through them with a mascara brush and dry them with a mini fan.

STEP 18

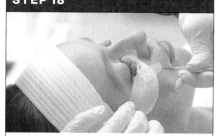

Remove the strips of tape first and then the eye pads to avoid pulling out any lower lashes that may be tucked between the pad and tape.

STEP 19

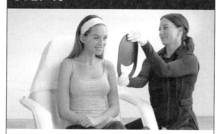

Show the client the finished look with a hand mirror and make sure the client is comfortable with the lashes.

POST SERVICE

Perform Procedure 4-4: Post-Service Procedure

Procedure 6-5: Eyelash Refill

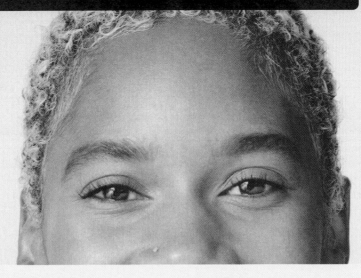

IMPLEMENTS AND MATERIALS:

- Adhesive remover
- Adjustable LED light
- Disposable lint-free applicators
- Disposable mascara brushes
- Disposable micro swabs
- Distilled water
- Eyelash cleanser
- Gloves
- Jade stone
- Mini fan
- Paper towels
- Squeeze bottle
- Surgical paper tape
- Trimming scissors
- Tweezers, curved
- Tweezers, straight pointed tip
- Under-eye gel pads

PREPARATION:

Perform Procedure 4-3: Pre-Service Procedure

PROCEDURE:

 30 MIN

BEFORE
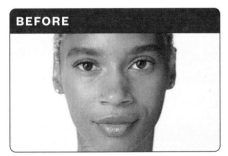

STEP 1
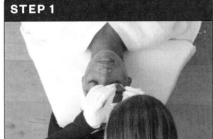

With the client lying down, use tweezers to examine the client's lashes and assess the extensions to be removed.

STEP 2
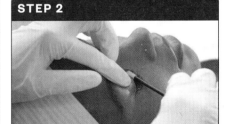

Cleanse the lashes in a downward motion using an eyelash cleanser and disposable lint-free applicators. Tilt the client's head to the side and, holding a folded paper towel to the side of their face, rinse with distilled water from a squeeze bottle.

Ch. 06: Eyelash Extension Application

Procedure 6-5: Eyelash Refill

STEP 3

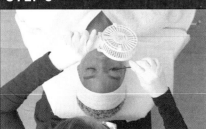

Gently pat the eye dry with the paper towel and repeat on the other eye. Thoroughly dry the lashes by brushing them through with a mascara brush and a mini fan, which will also remove any loose extensions.

STEP 4

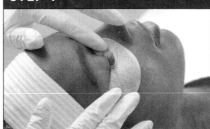

Remove the gel pads from their protective backing. While gently pulling back the client's eyelid, position the gel pads under each eye by covering the lower lash line. Be careful not to touch the inner eye rim.

STEP 5

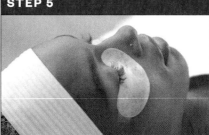

Cut two strips of surgical tape for each eye. Apply the strips under each eye by crossing them at the center of the lash line at a slight angle to cover any exposed lower lashes.

Tip: Always check in with your client to make sure the tape and pads are comfortable.

STEP 6

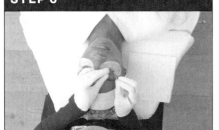

Locate eyelash extensions that have grown out and have extended beyond the 1 to 2 mm position in which they were placed or are peeling away from the natural lash they are attached to.

STEP 7

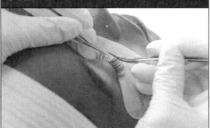

Using one set of tweezers, carefully grasp the natural lash and, using the other set of tweezers, grasp the lash extension. Gently peel the extension away from the natural lash, being careful not to tug on the natural lash. Place the discarded lashes on a paper towel for disposal in a covered trash can once you are finished.

Tip: If the lashes are difficult to remove by peeling apart, apply adhesive remover with a micro swab to remove and then cleanse the lashes before proceeding.

Caution!
If any adhesive residue remains, bonding of the new lashes will be compromised.

STEP 8

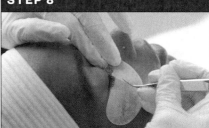

When you are finished with the lash extension removal, gently remove the strips of tape and eye pads.

STEP 9

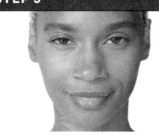

Proceed with the lash refill by following the technique for classic eyelash application or volume eyelash application.

POST SERVICE

Perform Procedure 4-4: Post-Service Procedure

Procedure 6-6: Eyelash Extension Removal

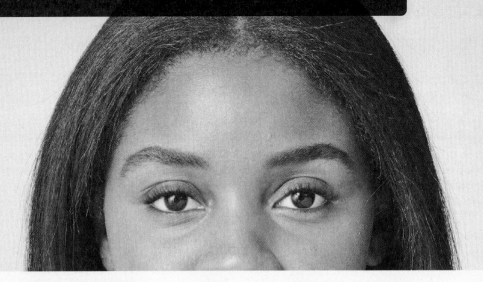

IMPLEMENTS AND MATERIALS:

- Adhesive remover
- Adjustable LED light
- Disposable cotton pads
- Disposable lint-free applicators
- Disposable mascara brushes
- Disposable micro swabs
- Distilled water
- Eyelash cleanser
- Gloves
- Jade stone
- Mini fan
- Paper towels
- Squeeze bottle
- Surgical paper tape
- Trimming scissors
- Tweezers, curved
- Tweezers, straight pointed tip
- Under-eye gel pads

PREPARATION:

Perform Procedure 4-3: Pre-Service Procedure

PROCEDURE:

30 MIN

BEFORE

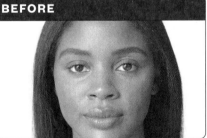

STEP 1

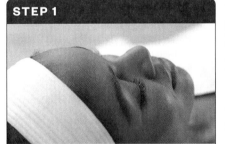

Ask the client to lie down with their head slightly inclined. This helps to prevent the adhesive remover from entering their eyes.

STEP 2

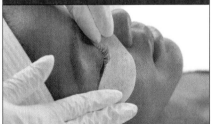

Remove the gel pads from their protective backing. While gently pulling back the client's eyelid, position the gel pads under each eye by covering the lower lash line. Be careful not to touch the inner eye rim.

Ch. 06: Eyelash Extension Application

Procedure 6-6: Eyelash Extension Removal

STEP 3

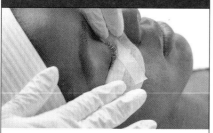

Cut two strips of surgical tape for each eye. Apply the strips under each eye by crossing them at the center of the lash line at a slight angle to cover any exposed lower lashes.

Tip: Always check in with your client to make sure the tape and pads are comfortable.

STEP 4

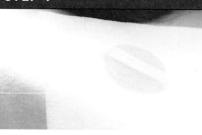

Cut two strips of surgical tape. Apply the strips by overlapping them on top of the jade stone or tile.

STEP 5

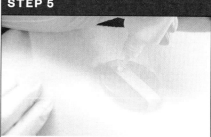

Dispense a small amount of adhesive remover onto the taped jade stone.

Caution!
If using a disposable lint-free applicator to dispense adhesive remover, always use a new applicator if more is needed during the procedure.

STEP 6

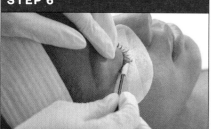

Apply adhesive remover using a disposable lint-free applicator in a downward motion and allow it to process according to the manufacturer's directions.

Caution!
Keep client sensitivities in mind when choosing the type of adhesive remover.

STEP 7

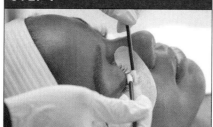

Using two new disposable lint-free applicators, gently stroke the lashes in an outward motion until the extensions are completely removed. Place the discarded lashes on a paper towel and dispose of them in a covered trash can once you are finished.

Tip: If needed, for single lash removal, apply a small amount of adhesive remover and wait two to three minutes. Use curved tweezers in your dominant hand to grasp the extension at the tip and pull back gently while holding the natural lash with straight tweezers in your nondominant hand.

STEP 8

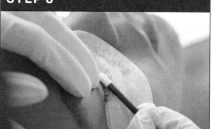

Cleanse the lashes in a downward motion using an eyelash cleanser and disposable lint-free applicators.

Procedure 6-6: Eyelash Extension Removal

STEP 9

Remove the strips of tape first and then the eye pads to avoid pulling out any lower lashes that may be tucked between the pad and tape.

STEP 10

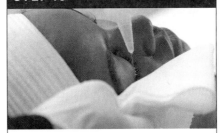

Tilt the client's head to the side and, holding a folded paper towel to the side of their face, rinse with distilled water from a squeeze bottle. Gently pat the eye dry with the paper towel and repeat on the other eye.

STEP 11

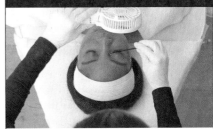

Using a damp cotton pad, wipe the lashes thoroughly. Dry the lashes by brushing them through with a mascara brush and using a mini fan.

Tip: If needed, apply fresh adhesive remover and cleanse and dry the lashes again until the client's lashes are completely residue free.

STEP 12

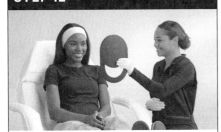

Show the client the finished look with a hand mirror.

POST SERVICE

Perform **Procedure 4–4: Post-Service Procedure**

Ch. 06: Eyelash Extension Application

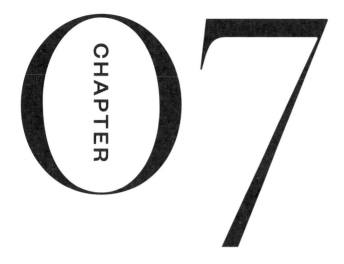

Eyelash and Eyebrow Chemical Services

🏳 Learning Objectives

After completing this chapter, you will be able to:

1. Explain the importance of understanding eyelash and eyebrow chemical services.
2. Demonstrate a thorough client consultation for eyelash and eyebrow chemical services.
3. Discuss the importance of aftercare for eyelash and eyebrow chemical services.
4. Perform an eyelash lifting (perming) application.
5. Perform an eyebrow lamination procedure.
6. Perform an eyelash tinting procedure.
7. Perform an eyebrow tinting procedure.

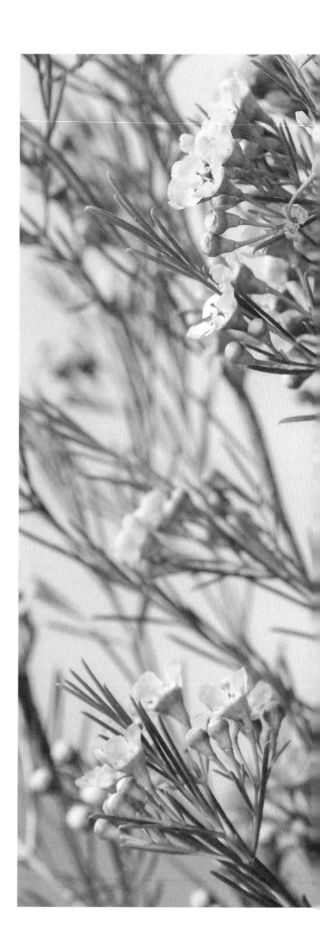

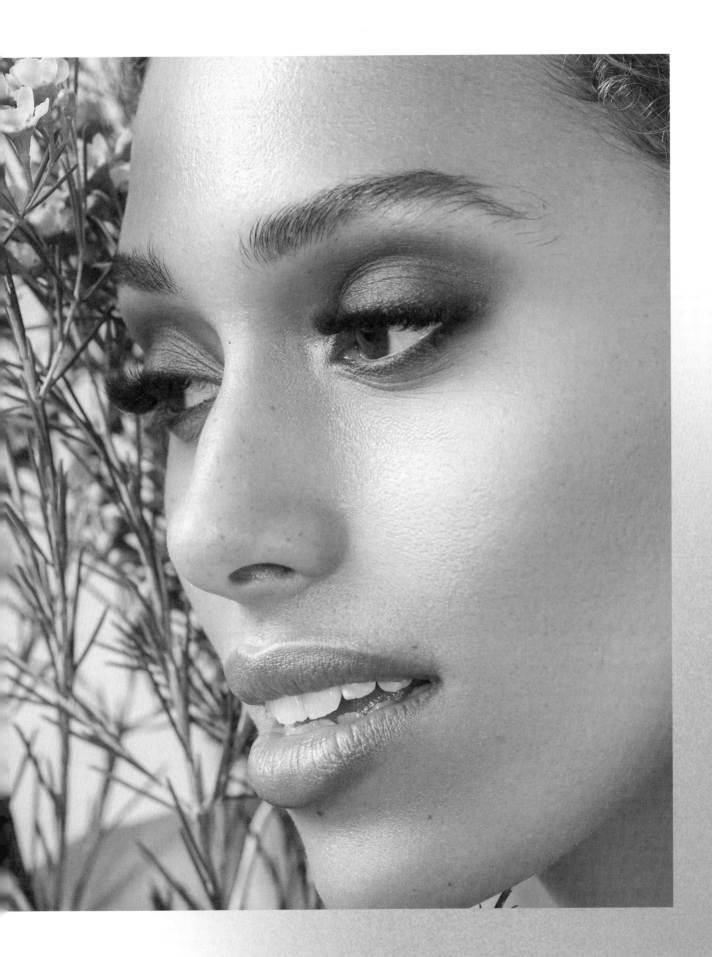

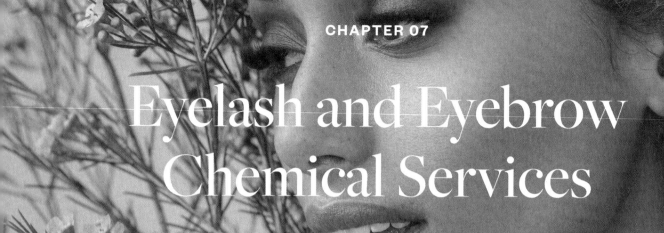

CHAPTER 07

Eyelash and Eyebrow Chemical Services

Why Study Eyelash and Eyebrow Chemical Services?

 Learning Objective 01

Explain the importance of understanding eyelash and eyebrow chemical services.

Eyelash and eyebrow chemical services are becoming a significant part of the beauty industry. Although these services can be draws in themselves, they also represent attractive add-ons to lash, skin, or hair services you already perform. Over the course of this chapter, you will learn proper eyelash lifting, eyebrow lamination, and eyelash and eyebrow tinting techniques that will quickly set you apart from other service providers. Learning the appropriate techniques needed for these services will boost your career by allowing you to offer top-tier services in your area.

Eyelash technicians should study and have a thorough understanding of eyelash and eyebrow chemical services because:

- Eyelash lifting, eyebrow lamination, eyelash tinting, and eyebrow tinting are popular services that naturally add on to lash, skin, or hair services.
- With highly visible results that last a relatively short time, eyelash and eyebrow chemical services encourage clients to rebook reliably and often.
- As chemical services, these procedures bring with them additional cautions when it comes to protecting your clients' skin and eye health.

 Check In

1. Why is it important to you to study eyelash and eyebrow chemical services?

166 Ch. 07: Eyelash and Eyebrow Chemical Services

Client Consultation

 Learning Objective 02

Demonstrate a thorough client consultation for eyelash and eyebrow chemical services.

As with all beauty services, the client consultation is a valuable tool to ensure safety and success for both you and your client. It provides the perfect time to clarify your client's needs and desires when it comes to the chemical service they've come in for, as well as to evaluate any contraindications that may make the service less effective or dangerous for them. See Chapter 6, Eyelash Extension Application, for much more on eye service consultations, including how to administer and work from a client consultation form **(Table 6-1)**.

 Caution!

Check with your state licensing division to see if eyelash lifting/perming and eyelash tinting fall within your scope of practice.

Once you have completed any client consultation forms and discussed your client's desired outcomes, you can begin making notes on your client's chart for the service ahead **(Table 7-1)**. These notes, which you'll complete after the service, will help you keep track of what chemical services your client has received, when they received them, how long they were processed for, etc. Mark the types of products you use and what aftercare products the client takes home as well.

Table 7-1   **Sample Lash and Brow Chemical Service Client Chart**

Name: _____ Date: _____

Service Performed: _____ Processing Times: _____

Kit Used: _____ Aftercare Products: _____

Tape: _____ Other Notes: _____

Lash Shield/Rod Size: _____

Ch. 07: Eyelash and Eyebrow Chemical Services

Contraindications

Contraindications for eyelash and eyebrow chemical services are very important to note during the consultation and to pay attention to throughout the service. Failure to communicate about contraindications can result in harm to your client, as well as an unsuccessful service. Many of the contraindications from Chapter 6, Eyelash Extension Application, apply to the services here, with the addition that the chemical solutions involved have their own safety risks, in some cases because they must contact the skin and cannot be isolated to the hairs alone.

 Caution!

If you have any doubt as to a client's sensitivity to a chemical you will be using in one of these services, perform a patch test 24 to 48 hours prior to the service time.

 Check In

2. Why is a client consultation necessary prior to performing eyelash and eyebrow chemical services?

....
....
....
....

Workbook Assessment

Fill in the Blank

Fill in the blanks below using words from the provided word bank.

QUESTION 1:

Like all beauty services, the .... is an important tool to ensure the success and safety for both the eyelash technician and their client.

QUESTION 2:

Vanya is consulting with a client who is at the salon for an eyebrow chemical service. This is the perfect time for Vanya to gain clarity on their client's desires and needs regarding the service, as well as to assess any .... that may make the service less effective or .... for the client.

Word Bank

after
harmful
skin
client
contraindications
when
chemical
client consultation
hair

QUESTION 3:

Rumi, an eyelash technician, sits with a client, completes the .... forms, and discusses the outcomes the client wants from a specific service. After that, Rumi makes notes on their client's chart for the service first and then completes the

notes .... the service. These notes help Rumi keep track of the chemical

services the client has received, ... they received them, and how long they were processed for, among other information.

QUESTION 4:

Contraindications for eyelash and eyebrow .... services are extremely

important to note during the .... and pay attention to throughout the service. Failure to communicate about contraindications can cause harm to your

...................., besides resulting in an ineffective service.

QUESTION 5:

Chemical solutions involved in eyelash and eyebrow chemical services have their own safety risks, because, in certain cases, they come into contact with the

.... and cannot be isolated to the .... alone.

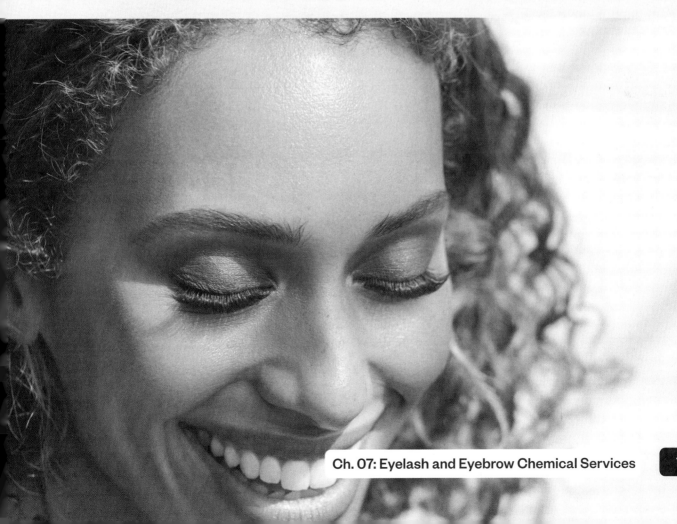

Ch. 07: Eyelash and Eyebrow Chemical Services

Client Aftercare

 Learning Objective 03

Discuss the importance of aftercare for eyelash and eyebrow chemical services.

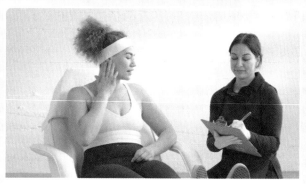

Fig. 7-1: Client aftercare is essential to creating happy customers.

Client aftercare is one of the most important things to discuss before clients leave your care, especially because you should never assume clients know how to care for their beauty services. Your client should walk away with full understanding of how to care for their services, as well as how long effects should last. Give them multiple opportunities to ask questions and clarify anything you've gone over **(Figure 7–1)**. Communication will build a healthy relationship with your client, creating happy returning customers.

Consider making and handing out aftercare cards to your clients and list aftercare protocol on your website to ensure your clients have access to these tips when they're needed. You should at least give your clients your contact information in case of an emergency or mishap.

Troubleshooting

No matter how proficient of a technician you are, there's a good chance that clients will come to you with questions about why their chemical service didn't last as long as they expected, wasn't as dramatic a change as they wanted, and so forth. In some cases, you may be able to do something immediately, such as reprocess a brow tint, depending on the previous processing time. In other cases, this troubleshooting will be an invitation to remind your client about proper aftercare procedures—for example, did they get their freshly laminated brows wet within 24 hours? Or perhaps to adjust your own procedures, such as doublechecking your calculations for how long to process hair of a certain texture.

Specific aftercare and troubleshooting tips appear in the procedure sections that follow.

 Check In

3. Who is responsible for the quality and longevity of your client's chemical service?

Workbook Assessment

Fill in the blanks below using words from the provided word bank.

Fill in the Blank

QUESTION 6:

One of the most important things you should discuss with your clients before they leave your care is client...................... You should never presume that clients know how to care for their beauty services.

QUESTION 7:

As an eyelash technician, you should ensure that your client leaves the salon after a service with a full understanding of how to..................... for the service and how long its..................... should last.

QUESTION 8:

When ensuring your client fully understands the aftercare required for a service, you must offer them multiple opportunities to..................... and clarify anything you have discussed..................... will help build a healthy relationship with your client, and it will lead to happy repeat customers.

QUESTION 9:

At Novo Salon, eyelash technicians hand out aftercare cards to their clients after each service. The salon also lists aftercare..................... on its website to make sure its clients have access to these tips at any time. Both the card and the website also include..................... for the clients in case of an emergency or any mishap.

QUESTION 10:

Clients are likely to come back with questions about why their chemical service did not last as long as expected, was not as dramatic a change as they wanted, and so on. Although in some cases you may be able to resolve their concerns immediately, in other cases, you will need to do..................... . It will be an invitation to remind your client about proper..................... procedures, or perhaps to adjust your own procedures.

Word Bank

troubleshooting
protocol
care
aftercare
communication
contact information
effects
ask questions

Ch. 07: Eyelash and Eyebrow Chemical Services

Eyelash Lifting (Perming)

> **Learning Objective 04**
>
> Perform an eyelash lifting (perming) application.

Permanent **eyelash lifting**, also called *eyelash perming*, involves the use of specially formulated products that keep natural eyelashes curled for long periods of time without the use of eyelash curlers. Permanent eyelash curling can make the eyes appear more open, giving the lashes a longer, more youthful look that lasts for several weeks **(Figure 7-2)**. When the permed lashes fall out and are replaced by naturally straighter lashes, the effect of the perming disappears. During the procedure, the natural lashes are adhered to shields or rods. A lifting solution, also called *perming solution*, is then applied to break the bonds of the eyelash hairs and form them to the shields or rods. This solution is capable of causing the hairs to stay curled for six to eight weeks. Once the solution is removed, a neutralizing solution is applied, which stops the perm solution from working, reforms the eyelash hairs, and sets them into the shape of the shields or rods. Post-treatment lotion can then be applied to nourish the eyelash hairs. Products should be used per the manufacturer's guidelines, as some brands vary. As always, safety is of the utmost importance. Using these products incorrectly can result in injury, chemical burns, or blindness.

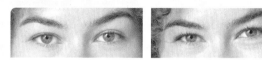

Fig. 7-2: Eyelash lifting creates an open-eye look.

> **Caution!**
>
> Perming solution for eyelashes and eyebrows is not the same as regular hair perming solution. The solution used for eyelashes and eyebrows is less potent and is a different consistency—typically a gel or cream—to control placement and stay out of the eyes.

Consultation

Ask the client to come in for a 15-minute consultation 24 hours before the application appointment. Examine the treatment area; if you see any redness, swelling, signs of conjunctivitis, or flaking, recommend that the client be seen by a healthcare provider or eye doctor prior to the service appointment. Clients with glaucoma, sensitivity to perming solutions, or thyroid conditions that affect hair growth are not candidates for eyelash lifting. Clients with recent vision-correction surgery should have clearance from their physician or wait until their eyes return to feeling typical.

To avoid an allergic reaction to the perming products, perform a patch test. Follow the manufacturer's recommendations for this process and refer any reaction to the client's healthcare provider. Do not perm lashes that appear weak or brittle. As with any products that you use on or near the eyes, be sure to follow the manufacturer's recommendations carefully. Failure to do so can result in ocular damage or blindness.

The consultation is also the time to discuss personalizing your client's lash lift. The shields and rods used in the lifting process can be customized for different levels of curl, ranging from more dramatic to more natural **(Figure 7-3)**. You will also want to select shields and rods that work best for your client's lash length and the shape of their eyes and eyelids. Also be on the lookout during the consultation for lashes that may be too short or sparse to effectively lift—these clients may be better served by eyelash extensions.

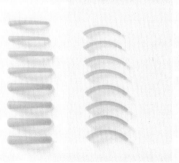

Fig. 7-3: Customize curl intensity by having a variety of lash shield and rod sizes.

Contraindications

Clients with the following conditions should not seek lash lifting:

- Pregnancy
- Excessive tears
- Eye irritations
- Eye infection
- Eye allergies
- Blepharitis
- Glaucoma
- Thyroid Conditions
- Recent eye surgeries
- Alopecia
- Chemotherapy
- Asthma

Clients with asthma may be sensitive to the odor of the perming solution.

Preparation, Health, and Safety

Advise the client not to wear mascara or eye makeup to the appointment. Removing mascara right before perming can irritate the eye. The client's contact lenses should also be removed prior to the procedure. Wash and dry your hands thoroughly and put on fresh gloves before starting the procedure.

Place your client in a reclined position on a disinfected treatment chair or table. Clean the lashes thoroughly with oil-free makeup remover and allow them to dry completely. This will ensure that the rods adhere to the lids.

Follow the steps for eyelash lifting (perming) in **Procedure 7–1: Eyelash Lifting (Perming).**

Perform:

Perform 7-1: Eyelash Lifting (Perming)

Perming with Other Lash Procedures

In some cases, clients may want to combine other services—such as eyelash extensions or eyelash tinting—with eyelash lifting. Unless otherwise indicated by a manufacturer, perform these procedures *after* you have permed the lashes according to the following guidelines.

- When adding eyelash extensions, wait a minimum of 48 hours after lifting the lashes to ensure that no residue from the perming solution remains on the lashes; be sure to use larger shields or rods to avoid overcurling. It is difficult to adhere lash extensions to tightly curled lashes.
- Eyelash tinting should be performed no sooner than 24 hours after eyelash lifting.
- Clients who have had permanent eyeliner procedures should wait a minimum of 4 weeks before any other procedures; the eyes need to be completely healed to avoid loss of lashes, irritation, and heightened risk of infection.

Aftercare

Make it clear to the client that they should not wet their freshly permed lashes for 24 hours. The lashes are still malleable within the first day, so it is important to inform the client that they should do their best to not sleep on their lashes within the first 24 hours. Sleeping on them can cause the lashes to alter their shape or crisscross over each other. You can also use this discussion to offer a retail product to add vitamins and nourishment back into the lashes.

Ch. 07: Eyelash and Eyebrow Chemical Services

Troubleshooting

Consider the following situations and their solutions.

- **Lashes aren't adhering to the shields or rods.** If you use too little adhesive, lashes won't stick **(Figure 7-4)**. You may also need to apply more glue than typical for stubborn lashes. Ensure that lashes are properly cleansed and free of debris that may cause interference. Lastly, check your adhesive product to make sure it hasn't expired and that you are storing it properly.

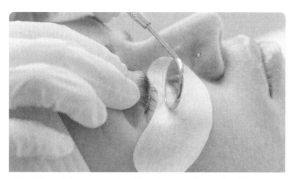

Fig. 7-4: Use enough adhesive to adhere lashes to the shields or rods.

- **The lift did not work, or the curl did not last.** There are multiple reasons that the lifting service did not work properly.
    - Check your products for their expiration date and proper storage.
    - Always start with properly cleansed lashes that are free of debris.
    - Using too much adhesive can prevent the lifting solution from penetrating the eyelash hairs. If needed, use the Y comb to remove excess solution.
    - Not enough lifting solution was applied to ensure adequate coverage of the lashes. This can happen when it is applied too thinly, when not enough of the mid-section of the lashes is covered, or when plastic wrap is used and smears the solution unevenly. Apply solution for adequate coverage and be gentle when using plastic wrap during processing.
    - The lashes were not allowed enough time to process. Check the manufacturer's guide for the appropriate processing time and use a timer during the service. If the client requests another service, it is safe to do so, keeping in mind the processing time you previously performed on the lashes.
    - Check in with your client on their aftercare routine!

- **Lashes are too curled after the service.** Make a note in the client chart to use a larger shield or rod at the next service. Overly curled lashes can be relaxed by gently combing the lashes with a mascara wand and lifting solution. Follow with neutralizing solution.

- **Lashes are messy or have an odd shape.** Crossed and messy-looking lashes occur when the lashes are not properly straightened on the shields or rods before processing and setting. After adhering lashes to the shields or rods, use the Y comb or eyelash separation tool to straighten and separate the lashes. If finished lashes have an L shape instead of a curl, the shields or rods were placed too far down on the eyelid. Ensure proper placement of the shields and rods before adhering the eyelashes **(Figure 7-5)**.

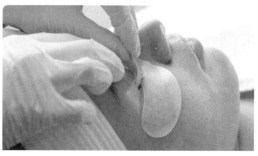

Fig. 7-5: Lash shields and rods should be placed as close to the lash line as possible.

- **Lashes are frizzy and damaged.** Do not allow the lifting solution or neutralizing solution to overprocess. Always follow the manufacturer's instructions for processing time. Frizzy lashes can also occur if the lifting solution is applied too close to the tips of the lashes, which are more delicate and process quicker. Remember to only apply to the midsection of the lashes.

Check In

4. How long does a lash lift last?

5. Can you tint lashes that have been lifted?

Workbook Assessment

Multiple Response

Please mark the correct answer(s) for each question. More than one answer may apply.

QUESTION 11:

Identify the features of permanent eyelash lifting.

- [ ] It helps keep natural eyelashes curled for long periods of time without using eyelash curlers.
- [ ] It is much like regular hair perming in that both services involve the use of highly potent solution that comes in a water-like runny consistency.
- [ ] It helps make natural eyelashes appear longer and thicker with the use of dyes that darken the lashes.
- [ ] It tends to make the eyes seem more open and gives the lashes a longer, more youthful look that lasts for many weeks.

QUESTION 12:

Diego has a consultation with a client who has made an appointment for eyelash lifting. What steps should Diego take during the consultation?

- [ ] Check whether the client has thyroid conditions that affect hair growth and, if yes, encourage them to perform eyelash lifting more frequently.
- [ ] Perform a patch test.
- [ ] Inspect the treatment area for any swelling, flaking, redness, or signs of conjunctivitis.
- [ ] Ensure that lashes that require lifting are actually weak.

QUESTION 13:

Identify some of the contraindications for eyelash lifting.

- [ ] pregnancy
- [ ] diabetes
- [ ] chemotherapy
- [ ] alopecia

QUESTION 14:

Zain is going to perform eyelash lifting on a client. Which of these steps should Zain take before starting the procedure?

- [ ] Ask the client to remove their contact lenses.
- [ ] Wear fresh gloves after washing and drying hands thoroughly.
- [ ] Make sure that the client's lashes are damp before starting the procedure.
- [ ] Clean the lashes thoroughly with an oil-based makeup remover.

Ch. 07: Eyelash and Eyebrow Chemical Services

QUESTION 15:

Maria is performing eyelash lifting on a client. They are facing difficulty with getting the lashes to stick to the shields or rods. Which of the following could have led to this issue?

☐ Maria used less adhesive than what was required.

☐ Maria applied the lifting solution too close to the tips of the lashes.

☐ The lashes are dry.

☐ The lashes have debris.

Eyebrow Lamination

 Learning Objective 05

Perform an eyebrow lamination procedure.

Eyebrow lamination has quickly become a leading service in the beauty industry. This service creates fuller, fluffy brows by using a chemical solution to groom the brows into a desired shape. Brow lamination is effective for anyone wanting fuller brows that are low maintenance **(Figure 7–6)**. Typically, clients will no longer need to fill in their brows with makeup after this service. Lamination is a great add-on, and results last 6 to 8 weeks.

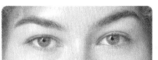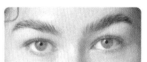

Fig. 7-6: Eyebrow lamination creates a full, fluffy brow look.

Eyebrow lamination is completed using three different products in three steps. These steps are typically purchased together as a kit. Each step is completed with a processing time determined by the health of the brow hairs and the texture they present with. Step 1 is a lifting solution that leaves the hair in the desired shape created by the service provider. After this solution processes, it is wiped off, and the next solution is applied. Step 2 is a neutralizing solution that stops the perming solution from working. It also holds the hair in the desired shape while the hair is smoothed. Once this solution is wiped off, the final solution is applied. Step 3 is a nourishing solution that calms the skin and puts vitamins back into the brow hair. Lamination can be harsh on the brows and surrounding skin. Be mindful when sharing proper aftercare and post-treatment recommendations with clients.

 Caution!

Be sure to check on your client and monitor their skin for reactivity. When it comes to sensitive skin, this service can be irritating. If your client expresses any discomfort, remove the solution with a wet cotton pad. Tingling is a common reaction; pain or intense stinging is not. This product *will* come into direct contact with the skin, so it is imperative to keep monitoring and checking on your client for a reaction or irritation.

Follow the steps for eyebrow lamination in **Procedure 7–2: Eyebrow Lamination.**

 Perform:

Perform 7-2: Eyebrow Lamination

Contraindications

Clients with the following conditions should not seek eyebrow lamination:

- Pregnancy or breastfeeding
- Irritated skin (acne, eczema, sunburn on the brows)
- Alopecia
- Recent permanent makeup procedures
- Use of retinols (includes Accutane), exfoliants using hydroxy acids (AHAs, BHAs)
- Very thin or short brows*

*Although clients with very thin or short brows may receive eyebrow lamination, they may not be able to get the results they desire.

Aftercare

Always look at the manufacturer's recommendations when going over aftercare. Advise your client to avoid getting their new brows wet for 24 hours. This will result in the lamination not lasting as long and losing the desired shape earlier. Nourishing oil is recommended for daily use. This will maintain the integrity of the hair, keeping the hair soft and hydrated. Advise your client to not sleep directly on their eyebrows for the first night. The hairs are very malleable at this stage and can take on an unwanted shape if slept on for a long period of time. Take this time to make sure to prebook your client out 6 weeks. These appointments are easy to forget about if rebooking is not completed.

If you have underprocessed your client, depending on their skin reaction, you may be able to reprocess the brows. Keep in mind your processing time, as well as how the brow hairs look. If they are starting to feel frizzy, it is not advised to keep processing the hairs. This will result in damage, breakage, or chemical burn.

> **Focus On**
>
> **Brow Styling**
>
> Show clients how to brush and shape their brows in the mirror before they leave the appointment. Brow lamination is very versatile, and brows can be worn however your client desires. Although some clients do not want their brows to look too full and fluffy, others specifically want that style. Make sure your client is aware of all options when it comes to styling their brows.

Troubleshooting

The chemicals used during a brow lamination can be quite potent. Advise your client to communicate if something is ever uncomfortable, burning, or stinging. A slight tingle is common, but anything beyond that means the solution should be removed immediately. Failure to do so can result in a chemical burn, damage to the hair, and discomfort to your client. To protect the client's skin around the eyebrows, apply petroleum jelly before starting the lamination process.

If the brow hair is extremely coarse or thick, a longer processing time may be necessary. As always, maintain communication with your client as to how their skin is feeling. Make sure the entire hair (down to the base) is saturated with the lamination solution. Specific hairs and areas of the brow may require a longer processing time **(Figure 7–7)**.

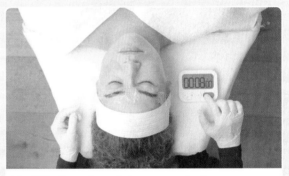

Fig. 7-7: Some brow hair may require longer processing time, but always check with the product manufacturer.

In case of underprocessing, the finished look will not be exactly what your client came for. Some brow hairs will lie neatly, whereas others stand up. It is safe to add more product and process longer if your client is still comfortable and the integrity of the hair and surrounding skin allow it. Communicate with your client regarding their service and how the hairs are responding. Booking more than enough time is important for this reason. As always, check the integrity of the hair and surrounding skin. Use your best judgement when processing the brows more than you already have.

On the flipside, brows that appear frizzy rather than full have been overprocessed. Do not process these a second time, as the problem will only get worse! These brows will likely need to be oiled, conditioned, and allowed to regrow.

Check In

6. What are the three solutions used in brow lamination?

7. Which type of reaction would promote removing the lamination solution in its entirety?

Workbook Assessment

Fill in the blanks below using words from the provided word bank.

Fill in the Blank

QUESTION 16:

.... services are used by clients to make the brows fuller and fluffy by using a chemical solution that grooms the brows into a preferred shape.

QUESTION 17:

Step .... of eyebrow lamination involves the use of a(n) .... solution that leaves the hair in the client's chosen shape created by the service provider.

QUESTION 18:

For clients with ...., the eyebrow lamination service is likely to be irritating. While .... is a normal reaction observed in clients, pain or intense .... is not.

QUESTION 19:

Clients with very .... or short brows are .... likely to get the desired results from eyebrow lamination.

QUESTION 20:

After performing eyebrow lamination, the technician should advise their client to avoid getting their new brows wet for .... as it could lead to the lamination lasting for a shorter duration and .... the desired shape earlier than usual.

Word Bank

sensitive skin

lifting

less; not

thin

24 hours (1 day)

safe

one

tingling

eyebrow lamination

losing

stinging

underprocessing

Ch. 07: Eyelash and Eyebrow Chemical Services

QUESTION 21:

After performing eyebrow lamination on a client, Lucas finds that the finished look is different from what the client wanted. They note that while some hairs lie neatly, others stand up. This is most likely to be a case of .... In such instances, it is .... to add more product and process longer.

Eyelash Tinting

 Learning Objective 06

Perform an eyelash tinting procedure.

Eyelash tinting involves the use of dyes to darken the natural lashes, making them appear longer and thicker. This service is great for clients who have light-colored lashes **(Figure 7–8)**. It allows clients not to worry about having to use mascara daily to darken their lashes and can last a few weeks. Keep in mind that clients need to have enough eyelashes to darken. If the client does not have enough eyelashes, they may be disappointed when it appears that tinting didn't work effectively.

 Caution!

Check your local and state laws for specifications on legal and safe tints. Tints using aniline derivatives (coal-tar based) can cause your client to go blind and are not approved by the Food and Drug Administration. Never use permanent hair color on eyelashes or eyebrows.

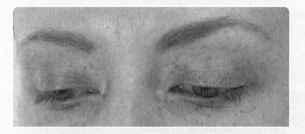
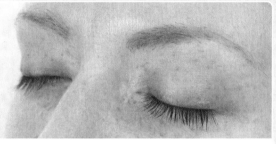

Fig. 7-8: Eyelash tinting will show the most effect on light-colored natural lashes.

Eyelash tinting involves the use of vegetable dye, semipermanent dye, or permanent. The consistency of tinting products varies. Vegetable dyes are usually fluid, whereas hair dyes are a thicker cream. The cream consistency provides more thorough coverage and is easier to apply consistently and precisely. Most lash tints are formulated using the same ingredients as hair dyes and come in a wide variety of colors, including black, blue-black, brown-black, brown, gray, blue, auburn, and chestnut.

Contraindications

Some situations indicate that eyelash tinting should not be performed. Clients with the following conditions should not have their lashes tinted:

- Pregnancy
- Blepharitis
- Glaucoma
- Eye irritations
- Eye infection
- Eye allergies
- Excessive tears
- Alopecia
- Very sparse lashes

Ch. 07: Eyelash and Eyebrow Chemical Services

Preparation, Health, and Safety

Before performing an eyelash tinting procedure, complete a consultation with your client. If sensitivities seem likely, perform a patch test. Make sure your client is comfortable and seated so that their head can be slightly reclined. Follow eye pad placement protocols (refer to Chapter 6, Eyelash Extension Application) to avoid getting tint on the skin.

Mix ¾ inch (2 cm) of tint cream with 2 to 4 drops of developer solution until the consistency is a creamy paste. Make sure that the consistency is not runny. Let the mixture set for at least 3 minutes while you prepare your client. For absolute accuracy, follow the product manufacturer's instructions.

 Caution!

If eyelash tint gets into the eyes, it can cause severe eye irritation or blindness.

Follow the steps for eyelash tinting in **Procedure 7–3: Eyelash Tinting.**

 Perform:

Perform 7-3: Eyelash Tinting

Aftercare

To ensure your client's tint lasts, instruct them to keep their lashes dry for a couple days, including no washing the eye area or wearing eye makeup during that time. Even after 48 hours, they should avoid swimming due to the chlorine. Hot temperatures, especially steam, should be avoided as well. Clients should also avoid sleeping on their face, rubbing their eyes, or using sticky strip lashes that can loosen eyelashes.

Oil-based products, including cleansers and makeup removers, will cause the tint to fade more quickly. Recommend that your client use a makeup remover for tinted lashes—these will often provide additional hydration and promote hair growth. Eyelash extension cleaners can be a good oil-free alternative.

Troubleshooting

If you or your client feel as though the tint did not process enough, it is safe to reapply the tint or use a darker color. Do not reapply the tint more than twice. Note the processing time on the client's chart to reference in the future. Check the product expiration date and that the product is properly stored.

 Check In

8. What type of products should clients with tinted lashes avoid?

Workbook Assessment

Multiple Response

Please mark the correct answer(s) for each question. More than one answer may apply.

QUESTION 22:

A client approaches Farah and expresses their wish to receive eyelash tinting, and they also ask for details about the procedure. Which of the following will Farah most likely highlight in their conversation with the client?

- [ ] This procedure will help the client avoid using mascara for a few weeks.
- [ ] This procedure is usually recommended for those who have sparse eyelashes.
- [ ] This procedure is great for those who have dark, long, and thick eyelashes.
- [ ] This procedure is recommended for those who have eyelashes that are light colored.

QUESTION 23:

Which of the following are true of products used for eyelash tinting?

- [ ] Eyelash tints come in two colors—black and brown.
- [ ] Eyelash tinting products include vegetable dye, semipermanent dye, or permanent dye.
- [ ] All products used for eyelash tinting have fluid-like consistency.
- [ ] Eyelash tints are usually made with the same ingredients as those used for hair dyes.

QUESTION 24:

Some of Klaus's regular clients have approached him to receive eyelash tinting. Which clients should receive the procedure?

- [ ] Tara, who is in the second trimester of pregnancy
- [ ] Yuji, who has a thyroid condition
- [ ] Paxton, who has light-colored lashes
- [ ] Dimitra, who has alopecia

QUESTION 25:

You have just performed eyelash tinting on one of your clients. What advice would you give the client regarding aftercare?

- [ ] Use oil-based cleansers and makeup removers.
- [ ] Avoid sleeping on their face.
- [ ] Ensure the eyelashes remain dry for the next 48 hours.
- [ ] Expose the eyelashes to steam.

QUESTION 26:
What steps should you take if a client complains that the eyelash tint did not process enough?

☐ Check the product expiration date.

☐ Use a darker color.

☐ Ask the client to wait for a week and make a new appointment for the procedure.

☐ Reapply the tint for as many times as needed to get the desired result.

Eyebrow Tinting

Learning Objective 07

Perform an eyebrow tinting procedure.

Eyebrow tinting is used to temporarily color brow hair **(Figure 7–9)**. The tints are the same as those used with eyelash tinting. As with eyelash tinting, tinted eyebrows allow people with lighter colored hair to have darker brows without having to pencil them in for a few weeks. Similarly, brow tinting is effective for those who have thick-enough eyebrow hair. Brow tint should only be applied to eyebrow hairs unless the client asks for their skin to be tinted as well. The tint will temporarily stain the skin if applied to it.

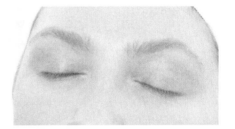
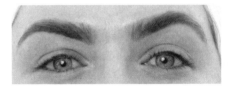

Fig. 7-9: Eyebrow tinting provides color and definition to eyebrows.

Preparation and aftercare for this service will be the same as eyelash tinting.

Follow the steps for eyebrow tinting in **Procedure 7–4: Eyebrow Tinting.**

P Perform:

Perform 7-4: Eyebrow Tinting

Ch. 07: Eyelash and Eyebrow Chemical Services

Contraindications

Clients with the following conditions should not seek eyebrow tinting:

- Pregnancy
- Irritated skin (acne, eczema, sunburn on the brows)
- Alopecia
- Very thin or short brows*

*Although clients with very thin or short brows may receive eyebrow tinting, they may not be able to get the results they desire.

Troubleshooting

Two common eyebrow tinting situations are:

- **Eyebrow tint gets on the client's skin.** Use a cotton swab to remove the tint from the skin before it can stain. Petroleum jelly can be applied to the skin surrounding the brows before beginning to preemptively protect it from staining.
- **Tint has stopped working.** Check your expiration dates and ensure you are using the correct ratio of tint color to developer. Always make sure that these products are stored properly.

 Did You Know?

When tinting unpigmented, gray hair you may need to use a darker shade and increase the processing time for good coverage. The amount of extra time needed will vary per client, so make sure to continually check to see if the color is dark enough before wiping away and to avoid overly darkening the hairs.

 Check In

9. Where can eyebrow tint be applied?

....

....

Workbook Assessment

Select whether the statements below are true or false.

True or False

QUESTION 27:

Brow tinting is effective for those who have sparse eyebrow hair.

T   F   why?..

QUESTION 28:

When performing eyebrow tinting, the technician should be careful to apply the tint to the skin rather than the eyebrow hair.

T   F   why?..

QUESTION 29:

Clients who are pregnant, have irritated skin, alopecia, or extremely thin or short brows should not seek eyebrow tinting.

T   F   why?..

QUESTION 30:

You should wet the client's brows with water before performing eyebrow tinting to preemptively protect the skin from tinting.

T   F   why?..

QUESTION 31:

Eyebrow tint works faster on gray hair.

T   F   why?..

Chapter Glossary

eyebrow lamination *AI-brau la-muh-NAY-shun*	p. 176	chemical service to groom brow hair into a fuller, fluffier shape
eyebrow tinting *AI-brau TIN-tihng*	p. 182	chemical service to temporarily color brow hair
eyelash lifting *AI-lash LIF-tihng*	p. 172	also called *eyelash perming*; chemical service to keep natural eyelashes curled for long periods of time without the use of eyelash curlers
eyelash tinting *AI-lash TIN-tihng*	p. 179	use of dyes to darken the natural lashes, making them appear longer and thicker

Procedure 7–1: Eyelash Lifting (Perming)

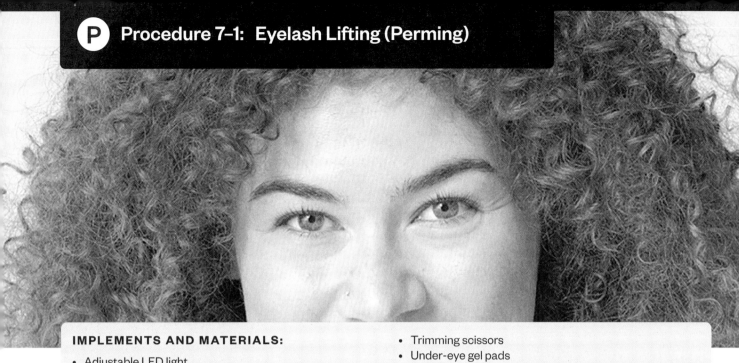

IMPLEMENTS AND MATERIALS:

- Adjustable LED light
- Assortment of silicone lash lift shields or rods
- Cotton pads
- Cotton swabs
- Dental mirror
- Disposable lint-free applicators
- Disposable mascara brushes
- Disposable micro swabs
- Distilled water
- Eyelash cleanser
- Eyelash separation tool
- Gloves
- Jade stone or adhesive holder
- Lash lift adhesive
- Lifting solution
- Mini fan
- Neutralizing solution
- Paper towels
- Plastic cling wrap (optional)
- Post-treatment lotion (optional)
- Single-use product tray supplied by the manufacturer in the lash lift kit
- Squeeze bottle
- Surgical paper tape
- Timer
- Trimming scissors
- Under-eye gel pads
- Y comb

PREPARATION:

Perform Procedure 4-3: Pre-Service Procedure

> **Caution!**
> Do not use hair perming solution on or near the eyes, as this can cause blindness and damage to the skin.

PROCEDURE:

 60 MIN

BEFORE

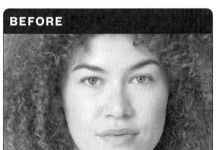

STEP 1

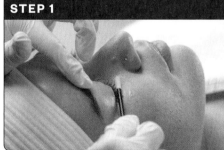

With the client lying down, sit behind them and cleanse the lashes in a downward motion using an eyelash cleanser and disposable lint-free applicators. Tilt the client's head to the side and, holding a folded paper towel to the side of their face, rinse with distilled water from a squeeze bottle.

Procedure 7-1: Eyelash Lifting (Perming)

STEP 2

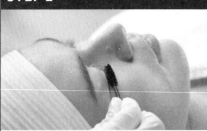

Gently pat the eye dry with the paper towel and repeat on the other eye. Thoroughly dry the lashes by brushing them through with a mascara brush and a mini fan.

Tip: If needed, repeat the cleansing process again until the eyelashes are free of residue.

STEP 3

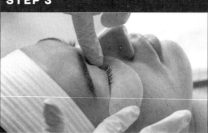

Remove the gel pads from their protective backing. While gently pulling back the client's eyelid, position the gel pads under each eye by covering the lower lash line. Be careful not to touch the inner eye rim.

STEP 4

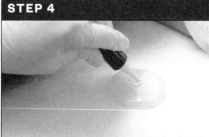

Cut two strips of surgical tape and apply them to the top of the jade stone or tile by overlapping them. Dispense lash lift adhesive onto the taped jade stone.

Tip: You will not need to dispense onto a jade stone if you are using a brush-on adhesive.

STEP 5

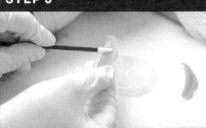

Select appropriately sized lash lift shields for the client's eyes. Apply lash lift adhesive with a lint-free applicator to the back of the shields and wait 10 to 20 seconds to allow the adhesive to become slightly tacky.

STEP 6

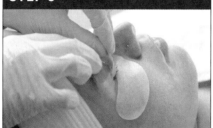

Place the shields as close to the lash line as possible without touching the lashes so they are able to curl around the shields comfortably.

STEP 7

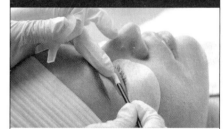

Starting at the outer corner, apply lash lift adhesive with a lint-free applicator on about 1/3 of the front of one shield. Work in sections to avoid the adhesive from drying too quickly.

STEP 8

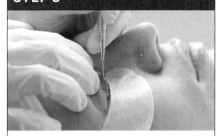

Once the adhesive is tacky, use the manufacturer's Y comb or an eyelash separation tool to flatten and straighten the lashes onto the shield.

STEP 9

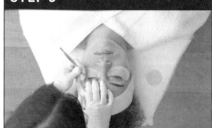

Repeat Steps 7 and 8 for the remaining sections until all lashes are flattened onto the shield. Repeat on the other eye.

STEP 10

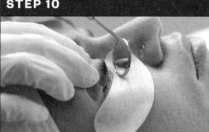

Using a dental mirror, check that all top lashes are secured to the shields and that there are no bottom lashes attached. Ensure top lashes are spaced across the shields without crossing over each other.

Procedure 7-1: Eyelash Lifting (Perming)

STEP 11

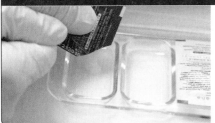

Dispense lifting solution into the single-use product tray supplied by the manufacturer in the lash lift kit.

Tip: You can dispense these solutions onto a jade stone (with tape or a protective sticker) and pick up with the lint-free applicators.

STEP 12

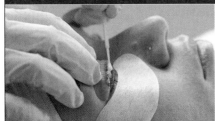

Apply lifting solution with a micro swab to the mid-section of the lashes, avoiding the base and tips. Follow the manufacturer's instructions for processing time.

Caution!
Do not let any perming solution enter the client's eyes or touch their skin.

Optional: Apply a small piece of plastic wrap over the top of the lashes to keep them secure and speed up the processing time. Use caution as this can produce excess heat.

STEP 13

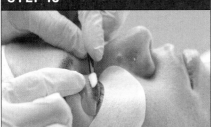

Gently remove lifting solution after the processing time using a lint-free applicator followed by a cotton pad. Follow the manufacturer's instructions for wet or dry removal is needed. Gently pat the lashes dry with a dry cotton pad.

STEP 14

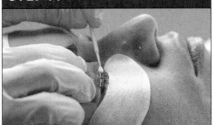

Dispense neutralizing solution into the tray and apply it with a new micro swab to the mid-section of the lashes, avoiding the base and tips. Follow the manufacturer's instructions for processing time.

Optional: Apply a small piece of plastic wrap over the top of the lashes to keep them secure and speed up the processing time. Use caution as this can produce excess heat.

STEP 15

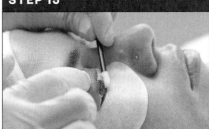

Gently remove the neutralizing solution after the processing time using a lint-free applicator followed by a cotton pad. Follow the manufacturer's instructions for wet or dry removal as needed.

Procedure 7–1: Eyelash Lifting (Perming)

STEP 16

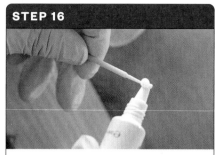

If the kit includes a post-treatment lotion, apply it with a fresh micro swab to the lashes. Let the lotion set according to the manufacturer's instructions.

STEP 17

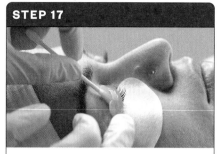

Release the lashes from the shield by using a damp cotton swab or lint-free applicator and swiping straight up from base to tips. Then, remove the shield from the eyelid by swiping a damp cotton swab underneath it and against the eyelid.

STEP 18

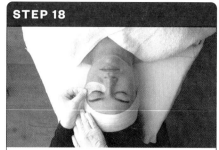

Remove the eye gel pads from under the eyes and clean the lashes with damp cotton pads.

STEP 19

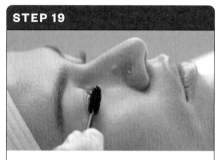

Brush through the lashes with a mascara brush and dry them with a mini fan.

STEP 20

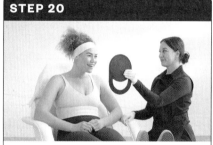

Show the client the finished look with a hand mirror.

POST SERVICE

Perform Procedure 4–4: Post-Service Procedure

Procedure 7-2: Eyebrow Lamination

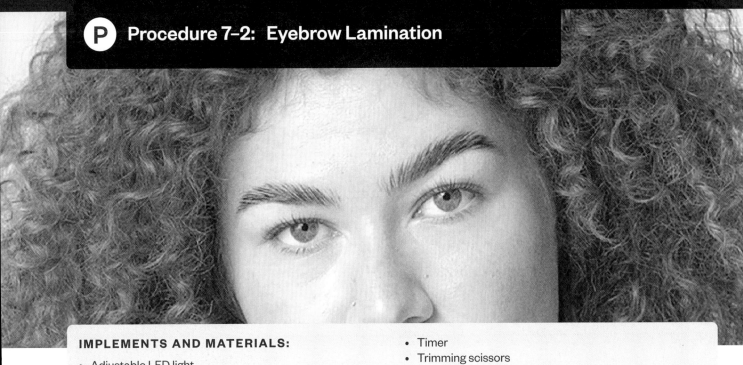

IMPLEMENTS AND MATERIALS:

- Adjustable LED light
- Cotton pads
- Disposable interdental brushes
- Disposable lint-free applicators
- Disposable mascara brushes
- Disposable micro swabs
- Distilled water
- Gloves
- Lifting solution/brow bonder
- Neutralizing solution
- Oil-free cleanser
- Plastic cling wrap (optional)
- Post-treatment lotion
- Single-use product tray supplied by the manufacturer in the eyebrow lamination kit
- Skin barrier cream or petroleum jelly (optional)
- Squeeze bottle
- Timer
- Trimming scissors

PREPARATION:

Perform Procedure 4-3: Pre-Service Procedure

PROCEDURE:

40 MIN

BEFORE

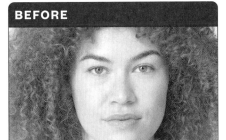

STEP 1

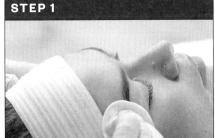

With the client laying down, thoroughly cleanse the client's eyebrows using an oil-free cleanser and cotton pads. Repeat if necessary.

Optional: Apply a skin barrier cream or petroleum jelly to the skin surrounding using a lint-free applicator for protection. If your kit uses glue, always apply skin barrier cream.

STEP 2

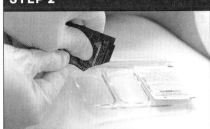

Dispense lifting solution into the single-use product tray supplied by the manufacturer in the lamination kit.

Tip: You can dispense these solutions onto a jade stone (with tape or a protective sticker) and pick them up with the lint-free applicators.

Ch. 07: Eyelash and Eyebrow Chemical Services

Procedure 7-2: Eyebrow Lamination

STEP 3

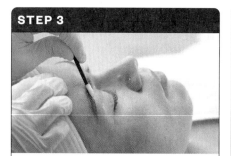

Apply a thin coat of the lifting solution to the eyebrow hair using a lint-free applicator or micro swab in the direction of the hair growth.

STEP 4

Slowly and carefully straighten and shape the eyebrow hair, setting it in the right direction, using an interdental brush or mascara brush. Follow the manufacturer's instructions for processing time.

Optional: Cover the eyebrows with plastic wrap. Use caution as this produces extra heat and speeds up processing time.

STEP 5

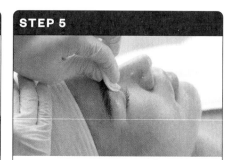

Remove the lifting solution using a lint-free applicator and then wipe with a damp cotton pad in the direction of the hair growth.

STEP 6

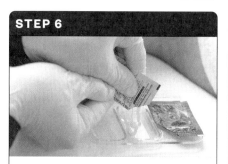

Dispense neutralizing solution into the tray and apply a small amount to the eyebrows using a lint-free applicator or micro swab in the direction of the hair growth.

STEP 7

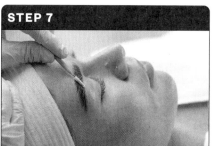

Brush brow hair into the desired shape, angling toward the temple, with an interdental brush or mascara brush. Follow the manufacturer's instructions for processing times.

Optional: Cover the eyebrows with a new piece of plastic wrap. Use caution as this produces extra heat and speeds up processing time.

STEP 8

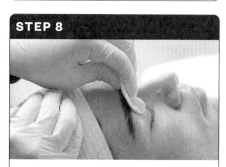

Remove neutralizing solution using a lint-free applicator and then wipe with a damp cotton pad in the direction of hair growth.

Tip: Depending on the product, the neutralizing lotion may be removed with a damp or dry cotton pad.

Procedure 7-2: Eyebrow Lamination

STEP 9

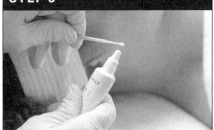

If the kit includes a post-treatment lotion, apply it to the brows using a new micro swab. Let the lotion set according to the manufacturer's instructions and then remove it with a lint-free applicator.

STEP 10

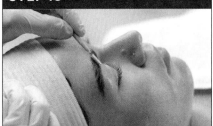

Brush through the brows using a mascara brush (interdental brush).

STEP 11

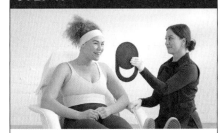

Show the client the finished look with a hand mirror.

POST SERVICE

Perform Procedure 4-4:
Post-Service Procedure

Ch. 07: Eyelash and Eyebrow Chemical Services

Procedure 7-3: Eyelash Tinting

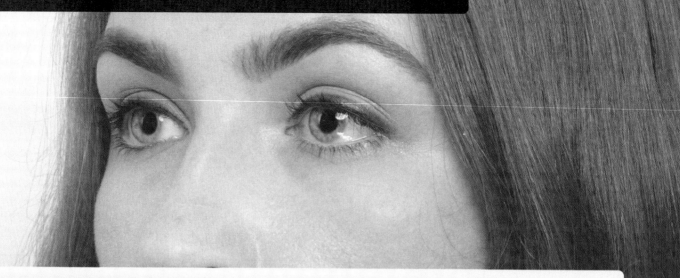

IMPLEMENTS AND MATERIALS:

- Cotton pads
- Cotton swabs
- Disposable lint-free applicators
- Disposable mascara brushes
- Distilled water
- Eyeliner brush (optional)
- Lash tint kit
- Oil-free cleanser
- Plastic mixing cup
- Skin barrier cream or petroleum jelly
- Squeeze bottle
- Timer
- Under-eye gel pads (or paper sheaths in tint kit)

PREPARATION:

Perform Procedure 4-3: Pre-Service Procedure

PROCEDURE:

 40 MIN

BEFORE

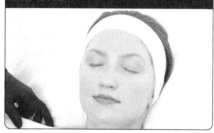

STEP 1

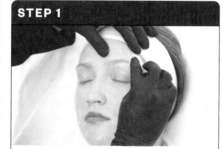

Cleanse the lash area. All makeup must be removed and the area must be clean and dry before applying tint.

STEP 2

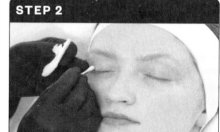

Apply protective cream on the skin below the eye and above the lashes, just next to the lash line, using a cotton swab.

Ch. 07: Eyelash and Eyebrow Chemical Services

Procedure 7-3: Eyelash Tinting

STEP 3

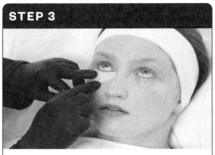

Apply pads under the eyes and over the cream to keep the tint from bleeding onto the skin. Alternatively, use the paper sheaths in the tint kit.

STEP 4

Ask the client to close their eyes, and adjust the pad so it sits next to the eye, not bunched up too close to the eye. If the pad is too close or too wet, the tint may wick into the eye and onto the skin.

STEP 5

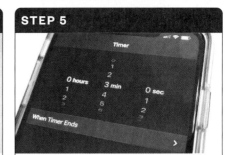

Prepare your timer according to the manufacturer's directions and have wet pads and cotton swabs ready to use for rinsing.

Tip: If you are also tinting the brows, you can start with the lashes and work on the brows while the lash tint is processing. Generally, the tint can sit on the lashes longer than the brows if you are going for a natural brow look.

STEP 6

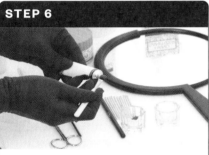

Prepare the tint. Place the amount of product you need into a cup-shaped palette.

Note: Some tint kits have only one bottle and combine the tint and developer into one application. If your kit requires the addition of developer to the tint, follow the manufacturer's directions for mixing.

STEP 7

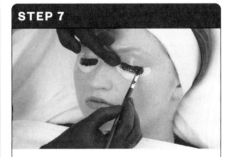

Apply the lash tint. Using a lint-free applicator or micro swab, apply the product from the base of the lashes to the tips. As another option, you can use an eyeliner brush, but be sure to properly cleanse and disinfect it afterward.

Note: Some manufacturers may suggest a second layer of protective sheaths that may be fitted over the tinted lashes at this time.

STEP 8

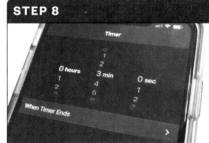

Begin the timer and leave the tint on as directed by the manufacturer's instructions. If your kit requires the application of developer in a separate step, use a new applicator to carefully apply the developer (bottle #2 for some kits) for 1 minute or as directed.

Procedure 7-3: Eyelash Tinting

STEP 9

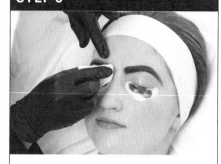

Rinse the lashes with water at least three times with wet cotton swabs and cotton pads without dripping water into the eyes. Have an emergency eyewash kit available in case any product gets into the client's eyes.

Tip: Before rinsing, you can replace the under-eye shields if necessary (if color is bleeding through the pads to the skin). Make sure the tint does not touch the skin.

STEP 10

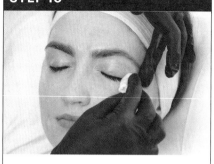

Remove the protective pads and continue to rinse the area thoroughly.

Caution!
To avoid eye damage, do not let the tint or water drip into the client's eyes. Ask the client to keep their eyes closed throughout the treatment.

Note: Ask the client if they feel any discomfort and help them to flush their eyes with water at the sink if necessary.

STEP 11

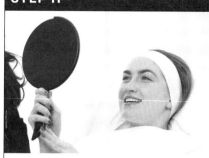

Using a mascara brush, dry the lashes. Show the client the finished look.

POST SERVICE

Perform Procedure 4-4: Post-Service Procedure

Ch. 07: Eyelash and Eyebrow Chemical Services

Procedure 7-4: Eyebrow Tinting

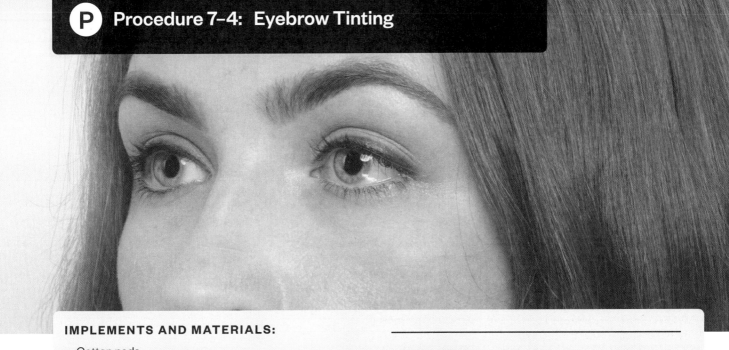

IMPLEMENTS AND MATERIALS:

- Cotton pads
- Cotton swabs
- Disposable lint-free applicators
- Disposable mascara wands
- Distilled water
- Eyeliner brush (optional)
- Brow tint kit
- Oil-free cleanser
- Plastic mixing cup
- Protective paper sheaths
- Skin barrier cream or petroleum jelly
- Squeeze bottle
- Timer

PREPARATION:

Perform Procedure 4-3: Pre-Service Procedure

PROCEDURE:

30 MIN

BEFORE

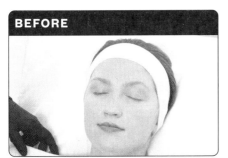

STEP 1

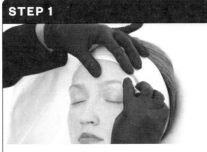

Cleanse the brow area and brush brows into place. All makeup must be removed and the area must be clean and dry before applying the tint.

STEP 2

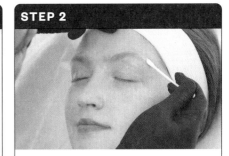

Apply protective cream with a cotton swab directly next to the area where you are tinting to protect the skin, covering the area where you do not want the tint. Do not touch the hairs with the cream because this interferes with the color. Apply the cream around the brow area.

Ch. 07: Eyelash and Eyebrow Chemical Services

Procedure 7-4: Eyebrow Tinting

STEP 3

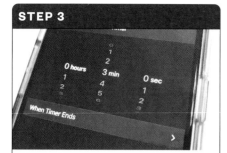

Prepare your timer according to the manufacturer's directions and have wet pads and cotton swabs ready to use for rinsing.

STEP 4

Prepare the tint. Place the amount of product you need into a cup-shaped palette.

Note: *Some tint kits have only one bottle and combine the tint and developer into one application. If your kit requires the addition of developer to the tint, follow the manufacturer's directions for mixing.*

STEP 5

Apply the brow tint. Apply the color from the inside to the outside edge of the brows.

> **Caution!**
> Brows can absorb color quickly, so be ready to remove it right away to avoid excess color.

STEP 6

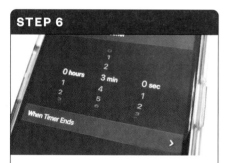

Begin the timer and leave on as directed by the manufacturer's instructions. If your kit requires the application of developer in a separate step, use a new applicator to carefully apply the developer (bottle #2 for some kits) for 1 minute or as directed.

STEP 7

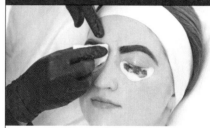

Rinse the brows with water at least three times with wet cotton swabs and cotton pads without dripping water into the eyes. Have an emergency eyewash kit available in case any product gets into the client's eyes.

> **Caution!**
> To avoid eye damage, do not let tint or water drip into the client's eyes. Ask the client to keep their eyes closed throughout the treatment.

STEP 8

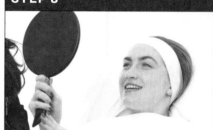

Using a mascara brush, dry the brows. Show the client the finished look.

POST SERVICE

Perform Procedure 4-4: Post-Service Procedure

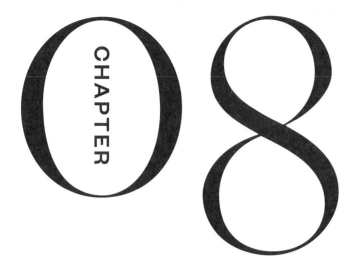

CHAPTER 08

Building an Eyelash Business

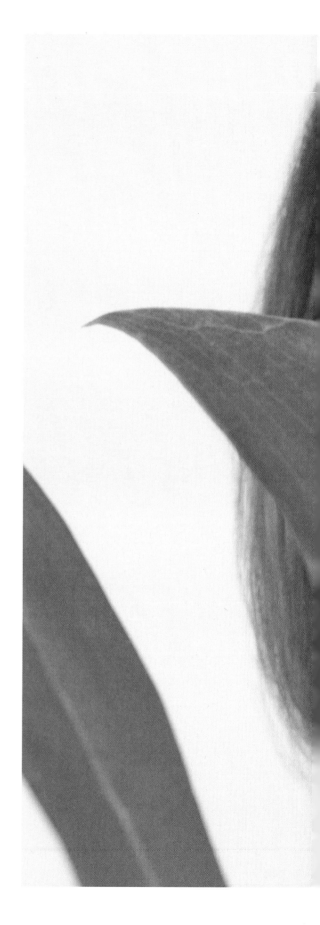

🏳 Learning Objectives

After completing this chapter, you will be able to:

1. Explain the importance of understanding how to build an eyelash business.
2. Discuss the impact of a professional image.
3. Define the role of ethics in business.
4. List the factors used to choose which products you buy.
5. Outline how to price services appropriately.
6. Identify how retailing affects your business.
7. Illustrate how to market your business to its full potential.
8. Describe how to utilize social media to your benefit.

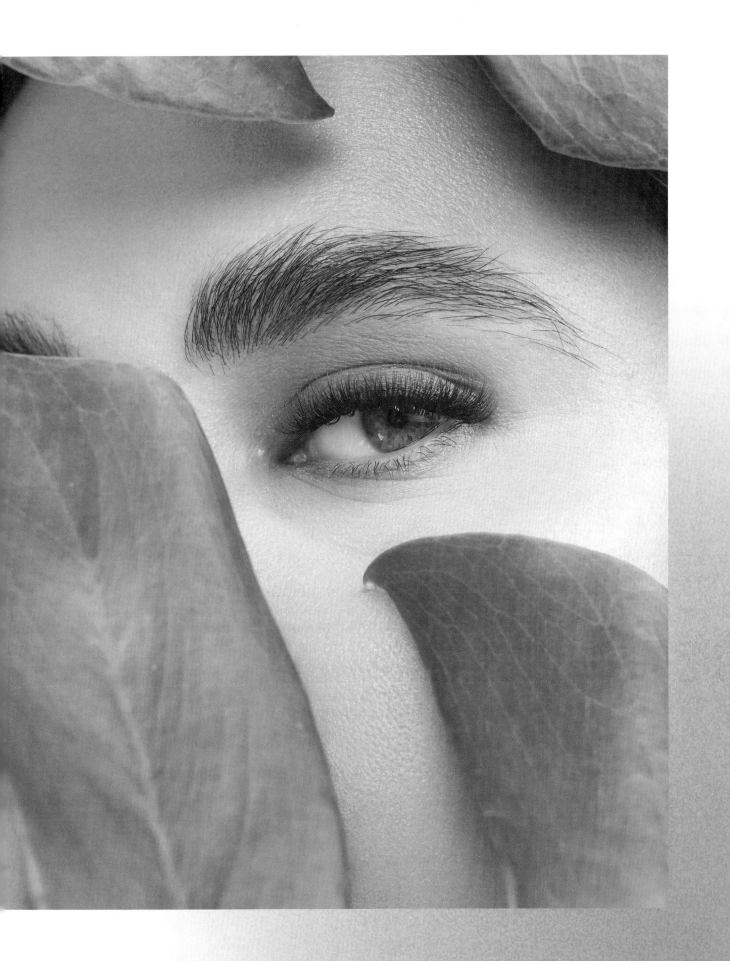

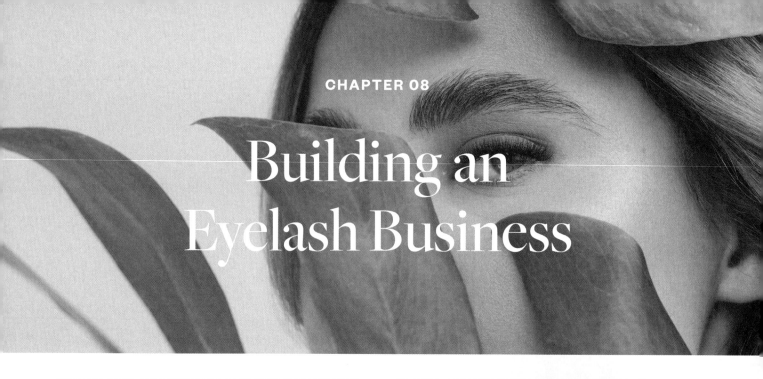

CHAPTER 08

Building an Eyelash Business

Why Study How to Build an Eyelash Business?

 Learning Objective 01

Explain the importance of understanding how to build an eyelash business.

As you continue to sharpen your technical skills, it's high time to think about your coming journey as a professional eyelash technician. It is not realistic to think you will be a celebrity lash artist right off the bat. However, building your clientele and perfecting your skillset is a step in the right direction. Be patient with yourself and your new skills. Success and confidence take time. It is important to take the necessary steps to run your lash business to maximize your income and set expectations that can be maintained throughout your career. This includes maintaining your professional image and brand, choosing the products that best fit your clients' needs, setting (and raising) your prices appropriately, and marketing yourself whenever and wherever possible **(Figure 8-1)**.

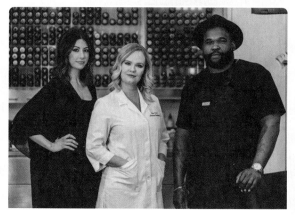

Fig. 8-1: Every opportunity is a stepping stone, so remember to look your best.

Eyelash technicians should study and have a thorough understanding of the business of eyelashes because:

- Your professional image is integral to how clients perceive your brand and colors their expectations of your skills and services. Your image is your best advertisement; make it a great one!

- Conducting business ethically, including communicating openly and honestly, should be a cornerstone of your eyelash career from the outset.

- You should feel supported and inspired by the products you choose to work with and retail. It is much easier to sell a product that you can talk about with enthusiasm and conviction.
- Marketing, especially viral marketing using social media, will be a major factor in your business's success or failure. What good are your amazing skills and boundless talents if nobody knows about them?

 Check In

1. Why is it important to you to study the business of eyelashes?

   ....

   ....

Professional Image

 Learning Objective 02

Discuss the impact of a professional image.

Your *professional image* is the impression you project through your outward appearance and your conduct in the workplace. Skill and talent may get you to the top, but it is your professional image and reputation that will keep you there, especially in the beauty industry. Would you go to a hairstylist who had bad hair? Or a nail tech who didn't have good nails? What about an eyelash tech who doesn't have great lashes? Looking the part is part of the job! When you are providing a luxury service, both established and potential clients expect a lot from your appearance and behavior. This includes how you act in public as well. Make it a point to always hold yourself to a high standard, as your potential clients are everywhere.

 Caution!

Salons and spas often have a no-fragrance policy for staff members because a significant number of people are sensitive or allergic to a variety of chemicals, including perfume oils. Whether or not your place of business has a no-fragrance policy, you should not wear cologne and perfume at work.

Personal Grooming

Appearance and personality are just as important as technical knowledge and skills. *Personal grooming* is the process of caring for parts of the body and maintaining an overall polished look. How a person dresses and takes care of their hair, skin, nails, and lashes reflects their personal grooming habits.

DRESS PROFESSIONALLY

While you are working, your wardrobe selection should express a professional image that is consistent with the image of your business **(Figure 8–2)**. Your clothes must be pressed and clean. Although some owners do not require their professionals to wear standard uniforms, they may have a specific dress code for the salon or spa. When shopping for work clothes, visualize how you would look in them while performing services. Is the image you will present one that is acceptable to your clients?

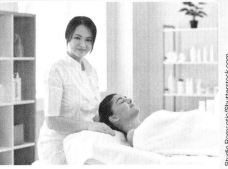

Fig. 8-2: Your work wardrobe should complement the image of your studio or salon.

Ch. 08: Building an Eyelash Business

MAINTAIN BEAUTY STANDARDS

Complement your professional wardrobe with an up-to-date hairstyle. If you wear a beard or moustache, be sure it is neat and trimmed; for the clean-shaven professional, shave daily if necessary and avoid undue stubble. Develop a skin care regimen that works best with your skin type. If used, makeup should enhance facial features, so take your time and apply makeup prior to arriving at work. Determine a nail length that suits your personal style and doesn't interfere with your ability to perform services.

Maintain your nails' appearance—broken nails or chipped nail polish may happen occasionally but should not be a regular occurrence.

In addition to the above beauty maintenance, it is in your best professional interest to ensure your lashes are on point as well. You are a walking billboard for your business; make sure great lashes are part of that advertisement. This carries even more weight if you wear a mask while working—with your mouth and nose covered, your eyes and eyelashes will be the stars of the show.

Personal Hygiene

Basic hygienic practices such as showering or bathing should never be omitted from daily personal care practices. *Personal hygiene* is the daily maintenance of cleanliness by practicing good, healthful habits. When working as a lash technician, you will by necessity be in close proximity to clients for long periods of time.

Focus On

Hygiene Packs

Create a hygiene pack to use at work. This pack should include the following items:

- Toothbrush and toothpaste
- Mouthwash
- Sanitizing hand wipes or liquid to clean your hands between clients (when soap and water are not available)
- Dental floss
- Deodorant or antiperspirant and body wipes

If you smoke cigarettes, do not smoke during work hours. Many clients find the lingering smell of smoke offensive. If you smoke during your lunch break, brush your teeth, use mouthwash, and wash your hands afterward!

Professional Attitude

Your artistic abilities and creativity are a gift; your attitude is something you can improve, polish, and continually develop to help you achieve success. The following actions can improve your professional attitude to keep referrals flowing and clients returning.

- *Improve your soft skills.* Being able to communicate will have the greatest impact on your career. Good speaking—and listening!—skills will allow you to communicate your vision to your client effectively and ensure that their expectations and needs are met. Successful communication between professional and client can be the difference between a satisfied client and success, or an unhappy client and failure.

- *Practice superior customer service.* Due to the nature of your profession, you will inevitably be providing a service for clients to purchase. It is up to you to provide every potential client with the best experience possible (**Figure 8–3**).

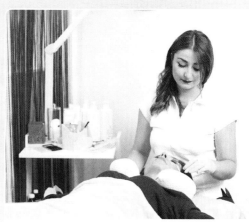

Fig. 8-3: Demonstrate your professionalism through exceptional experiences.

- *Be committed to an exceptional work ethic.* A solid work ethic incorporates doing what is right and being honest by staying motivated, displaying integrity, practicing good communication skills, and being enthusiastic in all of your endeavors.
- *Maintain time management.* Remember that you are responsible for your own time management. Sometimes, certain predicaments or instances arise that are unforeseen and unavoidable, and we do run late. If this happens, communicate with those who will be affected immediately—both clients and coworkers—and be prepared to offer solutions to make up for the lost time.
- *Remember continuing education.* The most successful lash technicians stay informed and up to date on the cutting edge of what is new and trending in their profession. There are many ways to stay informed and to gain the experience that will position you at the forefront of your contemporaries.

 Check In

2. Why is it important to maintain beauty standards, especially your lashes?

Workbook Assessment

Fill in the Blank

Fill in the blanks below using words from the provided word bank.

QUESTION 1:

.... is the impression one projects through one's conduct and

.... in one's place of work.

QUESTION 2:

Skill and talent may help an individual to get to the top, but it is the individual's

.... and professional image that will keep them there, particularly in the beauty industry.

Word Bank

personality
work ethic
professional image
communication skills
grooming
outward appearance
clothing

QUESTION 3:

Appearance and .... are equally important as technical knowledge and skills. The process of taking care of various parts of the body and maintaining a polished look overall is called personal ....….

QUESTION 4:

While working, an eyelash technician should ensure that their choice of .... conveys a professional image that is in line with the image of their business.

QUESTION 5:

Nora, an eyelash technician, maintains an excellent .... They make an effort to be honest and do the right thing by showing ...., remaining motivated, being enthusiastic in all they do, and practicing good ....

Word Bank

personality
work ethic
professional image
communication skills
grooming
outward appearance
clothing

Ethics

 Learning Objective 03

Define the role of ethics in business.

Ethics are the moral principles by which we live and work. In a salon setting, ethical standards should guide your conduct with clients and fellow employees. When your actions are respectful, courteous, and helpful, you are behaving in an ethical manner.

Practice ethical behavior on the job by employing these five professional actions:

- Provide skilled and competent services.
- Be honest, courteous, and sincere.
- Avoid sharing clients' private matters with others—even your closest friends.
- Participate in continuing education and stay on track with new information, techniques, and skills.
- Give clients accurate information about treatments and products.

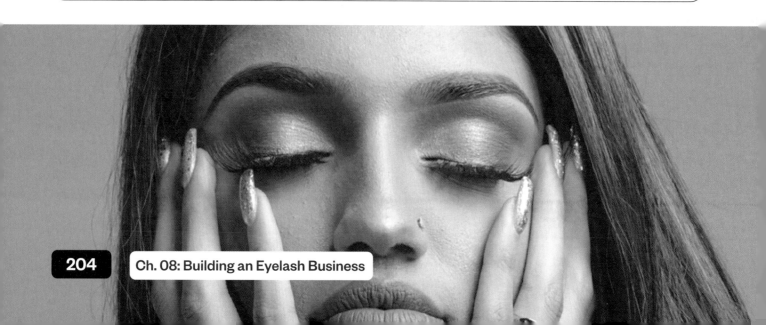

Ch. 08: Building an Eyelash Business

Professional Ethics

To be an ethical person, you should embody the following qualities:

- *Self-care.* To be helpful to others, it is essential to take care of yourself.
- *Integrity.* Maintain your integrity by aligning your behavior and actions to your values. For example, recommending products that clients do not really need is unethical behavior. On the other hand, if you feel that a client would benefit from certain products and additional services, it would be unethical not to give the client that information.
- *Discretion.* Do not share your personal issues with clients. Likewise, never breach confidentiality by repeating personal information that clients have shared with you.
- *Communication.* Your responsibility to behave ethically extends to your communications with clients and coworkers. Be aware of what you say and how you say it. Also, be conscious of your nonverbal communication, such as facial expressions and body language, which is just as important as verbal communication.

Ethical Communication

Open communication between you and your client is key when setting service expectations and building relationships. This means saying what you mean and meaning what you say, including not shying away from hard conversations. Listening to understand, not just with the intent to reply, is the other side of the coin. Keep in mind that a client who feels understood is more likely to take your advice.

When you have to turn a client away, do your best to educate and explain to your client why you can't perform or offer a service. Be precise to avoid being misinterpreted. Always do what is ethical for your reputation and the health of your client and their lashes. Jeopardizing the integrity of your service and business is not worth avoiding having a client feel sad or disappointed in the short term. Good communication skills can help ease these feelings or at least give some context for your client to understand.

See previous chapters for examples of contraindications that might cause you to decline a service, such as eyelashes that are too sparse or the presence of an infectious disease. Other situations that could push you to turn away a client include clients who want a style you don't or won't do, clients who are always late, or clients with chronically bad hygiene.

 Check In

3. What should you do if you have to turn away a client?

Ch. 08: Building an Eyelash Business

Workbook Assessment

Multiple Response

Please mark the correct answer(s) for each question. More than one answer may apply.

QUESTION 6:

Charlene is an eyelash technician. They have an exceptional work ethic and always exhibit high ethical standards. Which of the following are most likely to be true of Charlene's workplace behavior?

- [ ] They are respectful toward their clients and coworkers.
- [ ] They are courteous in all their interactions.
- [ ] They take the initiative to talk about their clients' lives with coworkers and close friends.
- [ ] They listen to clients with the sole intent of replying.

QUESTION 7:

Omar is mentoring Derek, a new eyelash technician at their salon. What advice should Omar give Derek regarding ethical behavior at the workplace?

- [ ] Omar should ask Derek to report everything the client shares with them to Omar.
- [ ] Omar should advise Derek to be honest and sincere in their interactions with coworkers and clients.
- [ ] Omar should advise Derek to refine their existing skills rather than focusing on acquiring new knowledge and skills.
- [ ] Omar should ask Derek to provide competent and skilled services to their clients.

QUESTION 8:

Which of these eyelash technicians embody the qualities of an ethical professional?

- [ ] Kristof, who avoids difficult conversations with their clients
- [ ] Kaia, who prioritizes self-care
- [ ] Lila, who refrains from discussing personal issues with clients
- [ ] Akira, who pushes retail products to clients who do not necessarily need them

QUESTION 9:

Which of the following are true of practicing ethical communication as an eyelash technician?

- [ ] It involves having open conversations with the client to establish expectations regarding services.
- [ ] It involves listening to the client with the sole intention of replying.
- [ ] It requires the technician to be precise in what they say to avoid being misunderstood.
- [ ] It requires the technician to avoid having difficult conversations with the client at all costs.

Ch. 08: Building an Eyelash Business

QUESTION 10:

Volga, an eyelash technician, is in a situation in which they must turn a client away. What steps should they take in the situation?

☐ Ask the client to leave the salon premises immediately.

☐ Ask a colleague to speak to the client in their stead and ask them to turn the client away.

☐ Explain in clear terms why the service cannot be offered.

☐ Avoid jeopardizing the integrity of the service even though it might disappoint the client.

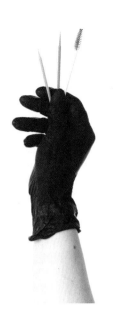

Choosing Products

 Learning Objective 04

List the factors used to choose which products you buy.

The task of adopting a line of products for service use or retail is a big decision. You'll be entering into a long-term business partnership and should expect to be supported in this relationship. Some questions you should consider when shopping for a product line include:

- Is the range of products versatile enough for your needs? Do they have all the lash extension lengths, curl sizes, and materials you want to offer?
- Are the ingredients used high quality?
- Does the manufacturer offer training and education opportunities for you to increase your skills?
- Do they provide business support, such as samples, brochures, marketing material, and favorable return policies?
- Are there minimum order sizes you will need to meet?
- Is the brand recognizable to clients when retailing?
- Is the packaging appealing and the product easy to use for client aftercare?
- Are the products sold directly to licensed professionals or can clients buy them directly online?

When evaluating the cost to you for service products, take the per-item cost and divide by how many months, weeks, or services the manufacturer says it should be good for. Use this number to compare products rather than simply the cost per item.

Aftercare Products

Aftercare is essential to the longevity of lash extensions. It is imperative that we over-communicate the importance of aftercare to ensure happy, satisfied clients. Selling a lash cleanser after completing a full set is both necessary and boosts your income with a product sale. Lash cleansers can be found within any lash brand, but it's important to choose one that you like, making it easier to talk about to your clientele. Ensure as well that any product you sell is lash safe. As most of the traffic you see will be lash extension customers, you need to be able to retail to these clients without compromising their lash health or longevity. For example, waterproof makeup is detrimental to lash extensions in any form. The oils present in waterproof makeup break down the bonds of the lash adhesive, making the extensions fall off quicker. Invest instead in an extension-safe product line.

Check In

4. What kind of support should you expect from a product manufacturer you buy from?

....

....

Workbook Assessment

Multiple Choice

Please circle the correct answer for each question below.

Ira is a senior eyelash technician at a salon. They are shopping for a line of products they need for different eyelash services and for retailing. They aim to enter a mutually beneficial long-term business relationship with the manufacturer of this product line.

QUESTION 11:

Which of the following questions should Ira consider when shopping for a product line?

A) Will the manufacturer give Ira a percentage of profits from doing business with the salon?

B) Does the manufacturer offer a versatile range of products?

C) Is the product line the least expensive one in the market?

D) Is the manufacturer open to using Ira's logo on their products?

QUESTION 12:

When shopping for a product line, what will Ira most likely do?

A) check if the manufacturer would give Ira a percentage of profits from the sale

B) compare products based on the cost per item

C) check whether the product is easy to use for client aftercare

D) check whether the product packaging design is consistent with the brand image of Ira's salon

QUESTION 13:

Ira has just completed a service wherein they applied a full set of eyelash extensions to a client. Which of the following will they most likely do after the service?

A) Ira will give a lash cleanser to the client as a complimentary gift.

B) Ira will recommend that the client use a regular facial cleanser to clean the lash extensions.

C) Ira will recommend that the client use only waterproof makeup for at least a week.

D) Ira will sell a lash cleanser to the client to ensure the longevity of the lash extensions.

QUESTION 14:

What should Ira do when buying aftercare products for lash extensions?

A) Ira should look for oil-based lash products.

B) Ira should select products that are popular on social media.

C) Ira should buy products that are safe for lashes.

D) Ira should ensure that the products they buy are waterproof.

QUESTION 15:

Ira plans to invest in a product line that is extension safe. This implies that Ira should do what?

A) purchase baby shampoo to clean lashes

B) avoid purchasing makeup products that are waterproof

C) purchase eyelash cleansers that contain sulfates and parabens

D) purchase alcohol-based wipes to clean their clients' lashes

Pricing Services

 Learning Objective 05

Outline how to price services appropriately.

Several factors influence the earning potential of an eyelash technician, from types of clients served, to types of lashes used, to frequency of appointments and geographic location. Your skill level and years of experience also determine your earning potential. How you run your business also plays a huge factor in your income. Not only do you need to provide a safe service, but you also must manage your business professionally. Depending on your employment situation, it's very likely that hours, income, retail, and nearly everything involved with being a lash technician are within your control!

For the most part, the cost of applying a set of lashes is relatively low. It is not the product the client is paying for, but your time and expertise. When determining your prices, don't be afraid to do some research and crunch the numbers:

- *Consider your costs.* On average, the total cost of products that go into a lash set is less than $25. This varies depending on the products your clients prefer or what you want to offer them. Whatever the consumable product cost to you, you should keep this absolute baseline in mind.

- *Check out competitor pricing and options.* Research within your area to see what services your competitors are offering and for how much **(Figure 8-4)**. You want to maintain your pricing close to the average rates (within $10 to $20) that are charged around you. Do your competitors offer event services (weddings, proms, etc.)? Decide if you'd like to compete for that as well and price accordingly.

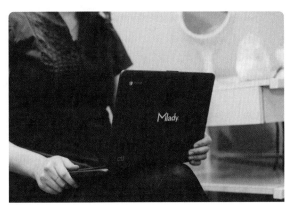

Fig. 8-4: Look up comparable services in your area to gauge your pricing strategy.

- *Determine client demographics and location.* Regardless of where you are located, lash extensions are considered a luxury service. However, your location and client demographics will affect what services you offer (are there high schools or universities nearby that would support graduation or prom services?) and how much you can expect clients to pay. Targeting a particular demographic can also help you set prices and offerings, as college students may not have the spending power or service expectations of an established professional working full time.

Even if you are new to lashing, do not undersell your services. As your timing gets better and your skillset starts to improve, raise your prices accordingly. Clients will value your increasing skills, and many will be happy to pay to keep them.

Getting to this level in your career takes time and should not be rushed. Practice makes progress, and it's important to not compare your experience to anyone else's journey along the way. We are working with tiny pieces of plastic, glued to a single natural eyelash. Be kind to yourself and give yourself credit for starting something new.

> **✓ Check In**
>
> 5. How should you price your services in relation to those of your local competitors?
>
> ....
>
> ....

Workbook Assessment

Fill in the Blank

Fill in the blanks below using words from the provided word bank.

QUESTION 16:

The earning potential of an eyelash technician is influenced by several factors such as types of .... used, types of clients served, geographic location, and frequency of ....

QUESTION 17:

The earning potential of an eyelash technician is determined by factors such as years of ...., their .... level, and the way they run their business.

QUESTION 18:

To a large extent, the cost of doing a set of lashes is relatively ....

The client is paying for the technician's .... and time rather than the products.

Word Bank

experience
average rates
expertise
baseline
skill
$25
low
lashes
appointments

Ch. 08: Building an Eyelash Business

QUESTION 19:

The total cost of products that go into a lash set on average is less than .... Regardless of the actual cost of the products used by eyelash technicians, they should keep this absolute .... in mind when pricing their services.

QUESTION 20:

When pricing services, an eyelash technician should research the pricing and options of their competitors. They must ensure that their pricing is close to the .... that are charged by their competitors in the area.

Retailing

Learning Objective 06

Identify how retailing affects your business.

Retailing product is a significant part of the business and an effective way to increase your income. Most salons will pay you 5 to 10 percent of every product you retail. Retail products, such as lash cleansers, lash accessories, skin care, body care, and brand-specific swag are always very popular. Maintain your retail area and make sure it is as place where people want to browse and spend additional time. Take note of expiration dates on all products you carry.

As a licensed professional, you will have access to both private label and commercial or consumer brands. Many national brands have programs for lash artists to receive a discount on the suggested retail price and are backed by quality assurances. Find a brand that you love, that you love to talk about, and that aligns with your values, then carry as much as you can from them. This will help you avoid ordering from multiple places at once. Consider the education and support that the company may offer as well. Knowledge is key when working with products that you will use and retail.

 Check In

6. How many brands should you plan to stock retail from?

Workbook Assessment

Select whether the statements below are true or false.

True or False

QUESTION 21:

Retailing product is often an ineffective way for eyelash technicians to increase their income.

T   F   why?..

QUESTION 22:

Salons usually pay technicians 35 to 40 percent of every product they retail.

T   F   why?..

QUESTION 23:

Retail products such as lash accessories, lash cleansers, body care, skin care, and brand-specific swag tend to be popular among clients.

T   F   why?..

QUESTION 24:

Several national brands have programs that allow lash artists to receive a discount off the proposed retail price of products.

T   F   why?..

QUESTION 25:

It is ideal for an eyelash technician to carry products of as many brands as possible at the same time.

T   F   why?..

Marketing

 Learning Objective 07

Illustrate how to market your business to its full potential.

Regardless of whether you collect a paycheck from an employer, are an independent contractor, or own your own business as an eyelash technician, *you* are your business. Your skills, abilities, professional traits, and success are completely dependent upon you. You are the one who builds, maintains, and grows your business. This is the power of the beauty industry: You have complete control over your growth, your success, and your business.

Branding Yourself

When starting out as a lash artist, it is important to think of your talent, skill, and professional image as a brand. Most artists find it difficult to "sell" themselves, so establishing your talent and skills as a cohesive brand will make it much easier and less intimidating to market and promote yourself. **Branding** is the character of your business and the personality and image you project to potential clients and employers. Everything clients and potential employers see must make a statement about who you are and what you offer. Use this to set yourself apart from other lash artists in your area. A logo is a unique symbol or design used to identify a specific organization or brand. If you have a logo, this should also reflect who you are as a professional. Make sure you choose something you can relate to and that is recognizable to potential clients.

Your logo, business card, website, portfolio, and social media—along with your professional image and work ethic—must work together to reflect, enhance, and support your brand throughout your networking and marketing efforts.

DEFINING YOUR BRAND

Defining your brand is a journey of self-discovery. It can be difficult, time-consuming, and uncomfortable. The image surrounding your brand is the principal source of your competitive advantage as a lash artist, and it is what will make you memorable.

The questions below will help you to define your brand:
- What do you want to be known for?
- What do you want your clients and potential clients to think of you and your work?
- What kind of message do you want your marketing to say to your potential clients?
- What can you do better than your competition?
- Why should people hire you and work with you?
- What sets you apart in an industry full of other lash artists?
- How do you provide a better service than your competitors?

Marketing Yourself

Marketing is how you convey your brand through promotions and advertising. Marketing sells your brand, and it is your brand that your clients will be attracted to and choose to buy.

Think of marketing as the method of attracting and retaining satisfied clients. It is the means for selling and promoting yourself. Your marketing efforts should effectively be 24/7 as you begin your lashing career. Marketing, however, takes time and patience. Just as the art of lash extension application requires diligence, so does marketing. Marketing will keep potential clients engaged in your business, so get up every day and put yourself out there.

Marketing has changed over the years and will continue to change as technology and buying psychology evolve. It is just as important to keep up with marketing advances as it is to keep up with the latest trends, products, and new innovations in the lash industry **(Figure 8–5)**.

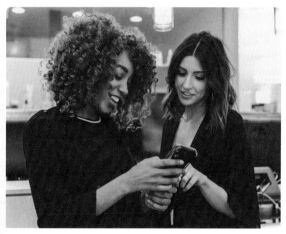

Fig. 8-5: Evolve your marketing plans as technology changes.

GETTING STARTED

Before you really start marketing yourself, you will need to have your website and portfolio ready for potential clients to view, as well as your social media pages. Even if you have very few photos and no clients, begin the process of creating these important marketing tools now as it takes time to research and develop what your brand will ultimately look like. Think of your bound portfolio, online portfolio, and website as your storefront. Remember that these are not only representations of your skills and talent but also of your professional image.

Nowadays creating your own website can be quick, easy, and quite fun. This is where you will send potential clients and employers to view your work. In addition to your work, you can post your resume to your website as well as behind-the-scenes photos and videos of you in your element. As with social media, only post photos and other material that represent you and your work in the best possible light. If it is not appropriate for all visitors to the site, then do not post it. Collect testimonials and referrals from clients and fellow technicians and post these to your website or portfolio as well. People will go to these places to find out more about you, what you can do for them, and how and if they want to contact you.

BUSINESS CARDS

Business cards are an important part of promoting business, and they help us swap information quickly and effectively. Create a memorable business card with your logo, website, or online portfolio information, phone, email, and social media handles. Tell the world what you specialize in and how good you are at it. Be creative, and hand out business cards everywhere you go—you never know where you will find a potential client. And remember, regardless of marketing ideas and money spent, the finest and most effective means of advertising is still word of mouth.

 Focus On

Marketing Yourself: Where and to Whom

A recent survey conducted by the Professional Beauty Association (PBA) yielded some informative results that all lash artists should keep in mind when planning marketing strategies. The top three ways that clients find a service provider, ordered from most often to least often, are as follows:

1. Recommendation/referral
2. Convenient location
3. Advertisement

The Number 1 thing you need to know if you want to grow your business in the shortest amount of time possible is: What are your clients telling their friends about you?

VIRAL MARKETING

The modern version of word of mouth is **viral marketing**, also known as *referral and recommendation*. It is personal communication about a service or product between target clients and their friends, relatives, and associates. The viral marketing technique passes along your message to hundreds and even thousands of potential clients through social media sites and email campaigns.

Viral marketing is a phenomenon named after the ability of viruses to act as infectious agents. In your case, these agents are clients who are so motivated about your services that they tell their friends and family, spreading your reach across networks, reaching into the thousands.

SOCIAL MEDIA

Social media will be your platform to engage and communicate with communities of people and is a great vehicle for viral marketing. Social media allows you to bridge geographical and cultural distances to reach a variety of people, usually with the same interests.

Social media for business is similar yet very different from personal pages you may have. It is a means to attract a following and have other people promote you and your business via viral marketing. Please note that it is recommended that you create a business page, rather than combining personal and business accounts. This will help you distinguish who you are speaking to and what your followers need to remain engaged.

As always, there will be people on social media who you cannot make happy. Keep in mind that these instances are rarely because of you! Always maintain professionalism and poise when handling negative comments or messages. If the situation is not being handled, feel free to leave it be. Be mindful that anything that is said/typed is public information, and you always want to appear professional if someone happens to screenshot what you wrote. *Remember:* It is most important to maintain professionalism at the times when it is hardest to maintain.

Marketing Ideas

There are many more traditional ways to market yourself as a professional lash artist and quickly establish a client base.

- *Advertising.* Place a small ad in a local paper, magazine, or newsletter around busy season, which starts in the spring.
- *Business cards.* Post your business cards at the local gym or fitness center. Consider leaving a business card with any bill you pay at a restaurant or coffee shop.
- *Establish relationships.* Nurture relationships with local hair salons, day spas, nail salons, and other establishments your potential clients could be frequenting **(Figure 8–6)**.

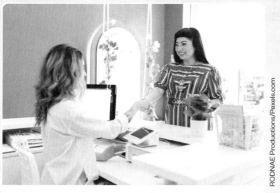

Fig. 8-6: Network with local businesses that share similar clientele.

- *Cross promotion with local businesses.* A very cost-effective way to market yourself is to partner with other local businesses in your area that share a similar client base to the one you service. Such businesses might include plastic surgeons, gyms, small clothing stores and boutiques, jewelry stores, Pilates studios, and so on.
- *Volunteer.* Perform complimentary full sets for local newscasters and television personalities. Perform demos or mini-classes at local cosmetology and esthetics schools and volunteer at women's shelters, local high schools, or career fairs.
- *Public relations events.* A great way to build your brand is to attend publicity events. Exposing your talents and skill to the public by getting the press involved can really get your name out among the public. Creating an effective and catchy press release that will attract the media's interest is important.
- *Chamber of Commerce.* This is a key one. Are you a member? Are you active? Again, low-cost networking involves being out in the community meeting and greeting people. Going to mixers or even being on the board has you connecting with like-minded people and generates exposure for you and your brand.
- *Local corporations.* Make a hit list of local corporations in your area—ones you want to target—and then call on them with an offering of a group VIP package for potential clients.
- *Charity events.* These venues create exposure, support a good cause, and get you connected with many people.
- *Free consultations.* If you currently offer hair, skin, makeup, or another beauty service, promote lash services as an add-on and sweeten the deal with a free consultation.
- *Gift certificates.* These are powerful tools in the business world. Gift certificates are a guarantee of additional revenue for the business. They are a great marketing tool to generate positive word of mouth.

 Did You Know?

Think about ways you can promote your talent. Dedicating yourself to a social media platform is a great method of creating a professional status and following that will help build your business. Post regularly—even every day—as it is well worth the effort and exposure. Potential clients will not know about your business or what you offer unless you tell them! Studies show that the average person needs to see an advertisement seven times before making the decision to become a client. Make sure you are staying relevant and showing your talent daily!

 Check In

7. What makes a good logo?

Ch. 08: Building an Eyelash Business

Workbook Assessment

Multiple Response

Please mark the correct answer(s) for each question. More than one answer may apply.

QUESTION 26:

Noah is a lash artist who is just starting out in their career. Which of the following should Noah do when establishing their brand?

- ☐ Ensure everything potential employers and clients see about Noah makes a statement about who Noah is and what they offer as a lash artist.
- ☐ Focus on building an image that reduces the differences between Noah and other lash artists in the area.
- ☐ Imitate the strategies of the most successful brands in the industry.
- ☐ Create a logo that reflects who they are as a professional.

QUESTION 27:

You successfully completed an eyelash extension certification course. Now you are thinking of creating a personal brand. Which of the following questions should you ask yourself to define your brand?

- ☐ How can I create a client base that rivals that of my competitors?
- ☐ What do I want to be known for?
- ☐ How can I make myself similar to my competitors?
- ☐ Why should potential employers hire me?

QUESTION 28:

Which of the following are true of marketing yourself as a lash artist?

- ☐ It is a method of communicating your brand through promotions and advertising.
- ☐ It is more important than building your brand.
- ☐ It is a one-time effort for attracting clients in the beginning of your career.
- ☐ It requires diligence, time, and patience.

QUESTION 29:

Identify the most common ways by which a client locates a service provider.

- ☐ anonymous reviews on online forums
- ☐ convenient location
- ☐ referrals
- ☐ door-to-door solicitation

QUESTION 30:

Jolene decides to establish a strong social media presence to market themself as an eyelash artist. Which of the following should Jolene keep in mind when engaging in social media marketing?

☐ Handle negative comments and messages in a professional manner.

☐ Share off-brand content frequently so that followers are updated on day-to-day life events.

☐ Distinguish between personal and business accounts on social media platforms.

☐ Avoid making multiple posts on the same day.

Social Media

 Learning Objective 08

Describe how to utilize social media to your benefit.

Social media has become a necessity at all levels of the marketing world. Harnessing this powerful tool will be key to helping you stand out in the saturated beauty industry. Most platforms are free and give you the capability of reaching thousands upon thousands of potential clients. It will be rare for you to meet anyone who is not on some kind of social media. Instagram, Facebook, Twitter, TikTok, and more are full of users who are looking for your services.

How to Use Social Media

All social media are platforms utilized to create an audience, showcase your work, and assist potential clients in finding you. The goal is that these followers begin to trust in your skillset, and eventually book an in-person appointment. The content posted on your pages should be directly related to the services you provide. Your name, colors, logo, and content should all fall within your established brand. For example, if you are a lash artist, you likely want to refrain from posting photos of your new shoes or what you are eating for lunch. The followers you have attracted to your page are following you to see your lash work **(Figure 8–7)**. You will notice followers losing interest if you go too off brand for their liking. Stay on brand and focus on your craft. Social media should also be treated as a form of customer service. If someone asks a question, sends you a direct message, or compliments your work, be sure to respond within 24 hours. Be kind, prompt, and professional in your response.

A number of social media sites exist that lash technicians can use to promote their brand through social media marketing. Popular sites and apps for advertising include Facebook, Instagram, Yelp, and Twitter.

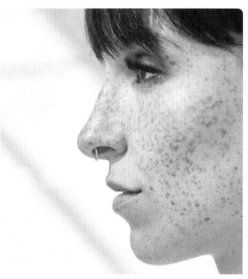

Fig. 8-7: Focus your business account on what clients want to see—your work!

When to Post

Social media can be a lot of work that can take a while to deliver its dividends. To start, the recommendation is to post once per day minimum. This sounds like a lot, but the more you post, the more relevant you'll stay on that platform. If this sounds unfeasible, start with every other day and work your way up to a daily post. Make it a priority to post at the same time every day. Wake up in the morning and post before you get up to shower. This habit will start to become familiar. Once this is a habit, ease into posting more and more. The goal is to post twice a day when you can, once in the morning and once at night. While you are building your audience, keep up that push to post often, and watch your business transform accordingly. Pay attention to the data collected to see when most of your audience is online and adjust post times accordingly.

What to Post

Figuring out what to post as a beginner lash artist can be challenging. Take photos of everything you do—yes, even if it's not your best work! Posting something is better than not posting at all. Post photos of your work, the instruments used to perform your job, your workspace, and most importantly, post you! Potential clients love to see what you look like. Share personal facts and information about yourself to gain the trust of your audience. If necessary, reuse photos you've already posted. Rotate the photo to look completely different. These are some tricks to utilize if you feel you have run out of things to post. All social media platforms are heading in the direction of favoring video content over still photos. Get comfortable being in front of the camera and putting yourself out there. Remember to be your most authentic self in this process. Potential clients who are watching should fall in love with who you really are and want to spend those long lash sessions with you. This will aid in creating happy clients that lead to lasting relationships.

Utilize social media to educate your audience. Whether it's about your services or about yourself, give them information they didn't know they needed. Create a blog, newsletter, advice column, or lash tip of the day. Tell them why you chose this career and what you love about it. Discuss your services, aftercare, and retail products, or even show the process behind what you are doing. Clients' eyes are closed for 90% of their appointment, so they never really get to see what you're doing. Show off your talents and confidence, in turn creating more trust with your current and potential clients.

Check In

8. Aside from marketing, how else should you use social media?

9. When should you make business posts on social media?

Workbook Assessment

Fill in the Blank

Fill in the blanks below using words from the provided word bank.

QUESTION 31:

.... has become essential at all levels of the marketing world. Most platforms are free and offer the ability to reach a multitude of potential ....

QUESTION 32:

Eyelash technicians can make use of social media platforms to build a(n) ...., showcase their ...., and help potential clients find them.

Word Bank

twice
social media
brand
audience
clients
customer service
work
one
related

Ch. 08: Building an Eyelash Business

QUESTION 33:

Donna, an eyelash technician, recently created an Instagram profile to attract potential clients. They should ensure that the content they post are directly

.... to the services they offer and that the name, logo, colors, and

content on the page are all consistent with their established ....

QUESTION 34:

Eyelash technicians should treat their professional social media pages as a form of

.... and be prompt, kind, and professional in their online interactions with existing and/or potential clients.

QUESTION 35:

When starting to create a social media presence for marketing eyelash services, it

is recommended that eyelash technicians make at least .... post(s) per day. Once this becomes a habit, the goal of eyelash technicians should be to post

.... a day when possible.

Chapter Glossary

branding **BRAN**-dihng	p. 213	the character of your business and the personality and image you project to potential clients and employers
viral marketing **VAI**-ruhl **MAAR**-kuh-tihng	p. 214	also known as referral and recommendation; the personal communication about a service or product between target clients and their friends, relatives, and associates

References

CHAPTER 01

1. Joyce Irene Whalley and Pliny, *Pliny the Elder, Historia naturalis* (1982).
2. Shannon K. Crawford, "How False Eyelashes Have Become a Must-Have, Everyday Accessory and a Booming Market," *ABC News,* May 8, 2018, https://abcnews.go.com/Lifestyle/false-eyelashes-everyday-accessory-booming-market/story?id=55019597.
3. Brandon Gaille, "33 Eyelash Extension Industry Statistics, Trends & Analysis," *Brandongaille.Com*, October 29, 2019, https://brandongaille.com/33-eyelash-extension-industry-statistics-trends-analysis/.
4. Ibid
5. The Business Research Company, "Personal Care Services Global Market Report 2021: COVID-19 Impact and Recovery to 2030," January 2021, https://www.researchandmarkets.com/reports/5238053/personal-care-services-global-market-report-2021.
6. Meghan Casserly, "Google to Glam: One Woman's Career Reboot Finds Cash in Lashes," *Forbes*, January 23, 2013, https://www.forbes.com/sites/meghancasserly/2013/01/23/google-to-glam-anna-phillips-thelash-lounge-entrepreneur/?sh=366dd5a94a5d.

CHAPTER 02

1. SOURCE: Bhupendra C. Patel, Michael J. Lopez, and Zachary P. Joos, *Anatomy, Head and Neck, Eyelash.* (Treasure Island, FL: StatPearls Publishing, 2022), https://www.ncbi.nlm.nih.gov/books/NBK537278/.
2. Erica Cirino, "Why Do We Have Eyebrows," healthline, March 1, 2018, https://www.healthline.com/health/why-do-we-have-eyebrows#Whats-the-purpose-of-eyebrows.

CHAPTER 03

1. Gary Clark, Sara M. Pope, and Khalid A. Jaboori, "Diagnosis and Treatment of Seborrheic Dermatitis," *American Family Physician* 91, no. 3 (2015): 185–190.

CHAPTER 04

1. U.S. Department of Labor's Occupational Safety & Health Administration, "OSHA QuickCard—Hazard Communication Safety Data Sheets," 2015, https://www.osha.gov/Publications/HazComm_QuickCard_SafetyData.html
2. Texas Department of Licensing & Regulation, "83.111. Health and Safety Standards—Blood and Body Fluids," *Cosmetology Administrative Rules,* October 20, 2020, https://www.tdlr.texas.gov/cosmet/cosmetrules.htm#83111.

CHAPTER 05

1. U.S. Environmental Protection Agency, "Facts About Formaldehyde," April 18, 2022, https://www.epa.gov/formaldehyde/facts-about-formaldehyde#research.
2. Editors of the Encyclopaedia Britannica, "Polymethyl Methacrylate," *Britannica,* December 4, 2018, https://www.britannica.com/science/polymethyl-methacrylate.
3. " Hydroquinone," *Wikipedia,* April 26, 2022, https://en.wikipedia.org/wiki/Hydroquinone.

References

4. American Osteopathic College Of Dermatology (AOCD), "Hydroquinone," 2022, https://www.aocd.org/general/custom.asp?page=Hydroquinone.

5. U.S. Food and Drug Administration, "Color Additive Status List," November 8, 2021, https://www.fda.gov/industry/color-additive-inventories/color-additive-status-list.

6. Wisconsin Department of Health Services, "Carbon Black," June 15, 2022, https://www.dhs.wisconsin.gov/chemical/carblack.htm.

7. "Silk vs Mink vs Synthetic Eyelash Extensions," *Secret Lash Paris,* May 14, 2020, https://secretlashparis.com/lash-secrets/silk-vs-mink-what-is-the-difference-and-which-one-is-better.

8. Mandy Jacobellis, "Choosing the Right Lash Extension Cleanser," *Lashx.Pro,* July 31, 2019, https://www.lashx.pro/blogs/lashobsessed/best-lash-cleanser-ingredients.

9. "Eyelash Extension Primer, Why Do I Need It?" *BL Lashes,* 2022, https://www.bllashes.com/blogs/blog/eyelash-extension-primer-retention.

Glossary

A

allergic contact dermatitis — p. 039 — an allergy to an ingredient or a chemical, usually caused by repeated skin contact with the chemical

uh-LUR-jihk KAHN-takt der-muh-TAI-tis

anagen — p. 030 — first stage of hair growth during which new hair is produced and actively growing

AN-uh-jen

asymptomatic — p. 064 — showing no symptoms or signs of infection

A-simp-toe-MA-tick

B

blepharitis — p. 037 — inflammation of the eyelids; chronically difficult to treat and causes dry eyes with occasional crusting or flakey material on the eyelashes after sleeping; commonly caused by staphylococcus

bleh-fuh-RYE-tis

boot tip tweezer — p. 092 — also called *L-shaped tweezer*; has a sharply angled curved tip and is mainly used for volume and mega volume lashing

boot tip TWEE-zur

branding — p. 213 — the character of your business and the personality and image you project to potential clients and employers

BRAN-dihng

C

carbon black — p. 088 — dark black powder used as a pigment; used as a coloring agent in adhesives

KAAR-bun blak

catagen — p. 030 — transitional stage of hair growth between active growth (anagen) and the resting stage (telogen)

KAT-uh-jen

chalazion — p. 038 — swelling or lump on the eyelid that is caused by the buildup of materials within a meibomian gland

kuh-LAY-zee-uhn

classic eyelash application — p. 132 — service in which single eyelash extensions are applied to single natural eyelashes

KLA-suhk AI-lash a-pluh-KAY-shun

cluster lashes — p. 130 — multiple artificial eyelashes grouped together at a short band or knotted base

KLUH-stur LA-shuhz

Glossary

conjunctiva *kon-juhngk-**TAI**-vuh*	p. 019	thin, clear, moist mucous membrane that coats the inner surface of the eyelids and outer surface of the eye
conjunctivitis *kuhn-juhngk-tuh-**VAI**-tis*	p. 037	also known as *pinkeye*; eye infection that may be caused by bacteria or virus; can be extremely contagious
contact dermatitis ***KAHN**-takt der-mah-**TAI**-tis*	p. 039	skin inflammation caused by contact with certain chemicals or substances
contraindications *kahn-**TRAH**-in-dih-**KAY**-shuns*	p. 124	situations in which eyelash extensions should not be applied because they could cause harm to the client
cornea ***kor**-nee-uh*	p. 019	transparent covering that protects the iris, pupil, lens, anterior chamber, and other internal structures of the eye; plays an important focusing role
curved tweezer *kurvd **TWEE**-zur*	p. 092	has a gentle curved tip and is typically used for isolation as well as precision placement of lash extensions
cyanoacrylate *sy-ah-noh-**AK**-ruh-layt*	p. 087	main component of eyelash extension adhesives; an acrylate monomer that is cured and used as an adhesive

D

demodex ***DEH**-muh-deks*	p. 038	contagious condition where microscopic mites burrow into and live inside the eyelash hair follicle; eyelash hair loss and potentially blindness
dry eye syndrome *drai ai **SIN**-drohm*	p. 039	lack of proper tear production, either because the tear ducts fail to produce enough tears or the tears evaporate due to physical problems with the eye

E

ectropion *ek-**TROH**-pee-ahn*	p. 039	causes the eyelid and lash to turn outward, usually the lower lids; involves loss of elasticity of the eyelid tissue and can require surgery to correct
entropion *uhn-**TROH**-pee-ahn*	p. 040	causes the eyelid to fold inward and the entire line of lashes to touch the cornea, which can scratch the cornea; involves loss of elasticity of the eyelid tissue and can require surgery to correct
exposure incident *ek-**SPOW**-zhur **IN**-sih-dent*	p. 064	contact with non-intact (broken) skin, blood, body fluid, or other potentially infectious materials that is the result of the performance of a worker's duties

Glossary

eyebrow lamination *AI*-brau la-muh-*NAY*-shun	p. 176	chemical service to groom brow hair into a fuller, fluffier shape
eyebrow tinting *AI*-brau *TIN*-tihng	p. 182	chemical service to temporarily color brow hair
eyelash lifting *AI*-lash *LIF*-tihng	p. 172	also called *eyelash perming*; chemical service to keep natural eyelashes curled for long periods of time without the use of eyelash curlers
eyelash refill *AI*-lash *REE*-fil	p. 137	procedure in which the outgrown eyelash extensions are removed and new eyelash extensions are put in their place
eyelash technicians *AI*-lash tek-*NI*-shun	p. 004	beauty professionals who perform eyelash extension services to enhance the appearance of the natural lashes while maintaining the health and integrity of the lashes
eyelash tinting *AI*-lash *TIN*-tihng	p. 179	chemical service to darken lashes
eyelashes *AI*-la-shuhz	p. 020	hairs at the edge of the eyelids
eyelids *AI*-lidz	p. 019	thin coverings of skin that protect the eye

F

formaldehyde fr-*MAL*-duh-hide	p. 088	colorless gas with a strong odor; a byproduct of curing cyanoacrylates

G

glands of Zeis *glandz of zees*	p. 019	sebaceous glands at the end of the eyelash follicle
glaucoma glaa-*KOW*-muh	p. 124	disease in which the optic nerve is damaged and can lead to progressive, irreversible loss of vision

H

hydroquinone hai-drow-kwuh-*NOWN*	p. 088	used as a stabilizing agent; keeps cyanoacrylate from curing in the bottle by stopping the polymerization process

I

individual lashes *in-duh-**VI**-joo-uhl **LA**-shuhz*	p. 130	separate artificial eyelashes applied one at a time on top of the client's lashes

L

lash fans *lash fanz*	p. 135	multiple single eyelash extensions grouped together with a single base and fanned out tips
lash map *lash map*	p. 120	guide for placing specific lengths of lash extensions in a set

M

madarosis *muh-duh-**ROH**-sis*	p. 040	loss of eyelashes or eyebrows, on one or both sides of the face
meibomian glands *may-**BOH**-me-uhn glandz*	p. 019	sebaceous glands at the back of the eyelid

O

ocular herpes ***AH**-kyuh-lur **HER**-peez*	p. 040	contagious infection of the cornea, the retina, or the uvea caused by the herpes simplex virus
ocular rosacea ***AH**-kyuh-lur row-**ZAY**-shuh*	p. 038	inflammation of the skin surrounding the eye, appearing as red, swollen, and highly sensitive eyelids or skin, possibly with broken blood vessels and acne-like bumps

P

polymerization ***PAHL**-uh-muh-ry-**ZAY**-shuhn*	p. 088	chemical process through which monomers form bonds with water to create long molecular chains; for example, cyanoacrylate turning from liquid adhesive into a solid glue
polymethyl methacrylate (PMMA) ***PAA**-lee-meh-thl muh-**THA**-kruh-layt*	p. 092	used as a thickening agent; a synthetic resin produced from the polymerization of methyl methacrylate

Glossary

R

round tweezers — p. 092 — have rounded tips that make it ideal for safely removing tape and eye pads after a service is completed

rownd TWEE-zurs

S

Safety Data Sheet (SDS) — p. 060 — required by law for all products sold; SDSs include safety information about products compiled by the manufacturer, including hazardous ingredients, safe use and handling procedures, proper disposal guidelines, and precautions to reduce the risk of accidental harm or overexposure

SAYF-tee DAY-tuh sheet

seborrheic dermatitis — p. 040 — skin condition caused by chronic inflammation of the sebaceous glands; often characterized by redness, dry or oily scaling, crusting, stubborn dandruff, and/or itchiness

seb-oh-REE-ick der-mah-TAI-tis

sensitization — p. 042 — allergic reaction created by repeated exposure to a chemical or a substance

sen-sih-ti-ZAY-shun

slant tweezers — p. 092 — typically used for eyebrow shaping; however, can also be used for applying temporary strip or cluster eyelashes

slant TWEE-zurs

sterilization — p. 057 — process that destroys all microbial life, including spores; requires use of an autoclave or flash sterilizer

steh-rih-luh-ZAY-shun

straight tweezers — p. 092 — long and narrow, ending in a tapered point ideal for picking up and placing lash extensions

strayt TWEE-zurs

strip lashes — p. 130 — also known as *band lashes*; eyelash hairs on a strip applied with adhesive to the natural lash line

strip LA-shuhz

stye — p. 038 — inflammation of a Zeis or meibomian gland that appears as a painful, red bump on the eyelid

sty

T

telogen — p. 030 — resting stage of hair growth; final phase in the hair cycle that lasts until the fully grown hair is shed

TEE-loh-jen

trichiasis — p. 040 — ingrowth of the lash, which can scratch the cornea

try-KY-uh-sis

V

viral marketing *VAI*-ruhl *MAAR*-kuh-tihng	p. 214	also known as referral and recommendation; the personal communication about a service or product between target clients and their friends, relatives, and associates
volume eyelash application vol-*YOOM AI*-lash a-pluh-*KAY*-shun	p. 135	service in which eyelash extensions are made into lash fans and applied to single natural eyelashes

Index

Note: Page numbers followed by f and t represent figures and tables respectively.

A

Accidental release measures, 62
Adhesives
    eyelash extension adhesive
        carbon black, 88
        cyanoacrylate, 87
        drying *vs.* curing, 88, 88f
        formaldehyde, 88
        humidity and temperature, 89
        hydroquinone, 88
        polymethyl methacrylate, 88
        storage, 89
    patch tests, 44, 44f
    skin reactions from
        dyes, 43
        latex, 43
    temporary eyelash adhesive, 90, 90f
Adhesive stickers, 95
Adjustable light or magnifying light glasses, 96
Advertising, 219
Aftercare product line, 211
Allergic conjunctivitis, 37, 37f
Allergic contact dermatitis, 39
Allergy *vs.* sensitivity. *See also* Disorders and diseases of eye area
    patch tests, 44
    sensitization, 42
    skin reactions, reasons for, 42–43
Almond eyes, 23t
Anagen stage, eyelash hair growth, 30
Anatomy
    of eye, 19, 19f
    of eyebrows, 20, 20f
    of eyelashes, 20
    of eyelids, 19, 19f
    workbook assessment, 21–22
Antibacterial soaps, 54
Aqueous humor, 19
Artificial eyebrows/eyelashes
    made by Karl Nessler, 7t
Artificial lashes, 4
    application of, 30
    invented by Anna Taylor, 7t
    made with thin plastic, 7t
Asymptomatic clients, 64
Autoclave, 96

B

Banana peel method, 140
Beauty standards, maintaining, 206
Blepharitis, 37, 37f
Blood exposure, 64
Boot tip tweezer, 92
Branding, 217
Bulbar conjunctiva. *See* Ocular conjunctiva
Bulb syringe, 94
Business cards, 218, 219
Butyl-Cyanoacrylate, 87

C

Carbon black, 43, 88
Carcinogen, 62
Catagen stage, eyelash hair growth, 30
Cat-eye lash map, 121, 121f
Celebrity, influence on eyelash products, 7
Chalazion, 38, 38f
Chamber of Commerce, 219
Charity events, 219
Chemical removers, 140
Chemical services
    client aftercare, 173–174, 173f
    client consultation, 171–172, 171t
    eyebrow lamination
        aftercare, 180–181
        contraindications, 180
        procedure, 180, 193–195
        troubleshooting, 181, 181f
    eyebrow tinting
        about, 186, 186f
        contraindications, 187
        procedure for, 199–200
        troubleshooting, 187
    eyelash lifting
        aftercare, 177
        consultation, 176, 176f
        contraindications, 177
        other lash procedures, 177
        preparation, health, and safety, 177
        troubleshooting, 177–178, 177f
    eyelash tinting
        aftercare, 184
        contraindications, 183
        preparation, health, and safety, 184
        procedure for, 183, 183f, 196–198
        troubleshooting, 184
    overview, 170
    workbook assessment, 172–173, 174–175, 179–180, 182–183, 185–186, 187–188
Chemical sunscreen, as allergen, 42
Classic eyelash application, 132, 132f
    application variation, 132
    lash extension placement, 132
    procedure for, 132, 153–155
Classic lashes, 118

Index

Claustrophobic clients, 124
Cleaning and disinfecting
    clean towels and linens, 57
    disinfectant log, 60t
    disinfectant tips and safety, 59, 59f
    disinfecting equipment, 57
    disinfecting work surfaces, 57
    multiuse products, 58
    nonporous, reusable items, 56, 56f, 71–72
    safety data sheet (SDS), 60–62, 60f, 61f
    sterilizers, 57, 57f
    of treatment area, 58
Clean towels and linens, 57
Client aftercare, 142–143, 143f, 173–174, 173f
Client consultation, 171–172, 171t
    consultation form, 114, 114f–115f
    preparing client for, 113
Client demographics and location, 213
Client headbands, 94
Client injury, 80–81
Client safety and infection control, 50–83
    cleaning and disinfecting
        clean towels and linens, 57
        disinfectant log, 60t
        disinfectant tips and safety, 59, 59f
        disinfecting equipment, 57
        disinfecting work surfaces, 57
        multiuse products, 58
        nonporous, reusable items, 56, 56f, 71–72
        safety data sheet (SDS), 60–62, 60f, 61f
        sterilizers, 57, 57f
        of treatment area, 58
    client injury, 80–81
    employee injury, 82–83
    exposure incidents
        blood exposure, 64
        eyewash stations, 65
        personal protective equipment, 65
        standard precautions, 64
    hand washing, 53, 69–70
        antibacterial soaps, 54
        waterless hand sanitizers, 54
    hygiene standard, 51
    personal habits, 51
    post-service procedure, 77–79
    pre-service procedure, 73–76
    prevention, 51
    workbook assessment, 52–53, 55, 63, 66–67
Close set eyes, 25t
Cluster lashes, 130, 150–152
Combustible material, 62
Commitment to work ethic, 207
Communication, ethical, 209
Competitor pricing, 213

Complete immersion, 56
Conjunctiva, 19
Conjunctivitis
    allergic, 37, 37f
    bacterial or viral, 37
    symptoms, 37
    treatment of, 37
Contact dermatitis
    allergic, 39
    irritant, 39, 39f
Contact lenses, 124
Cornea, 19
Cosmetics, in Victorian Era, 6
Cost estimation, 213
Cross promotion with local businesses, 219
Curved tweezer, 92
Customer service, improving, 206
Cyanoacrylate, 87
    in adhesives, 43

D

Deep set eyes, 25t
Demodex, 38, 38f
Diamond face shape, 26t
Disinfectant log, 60t
Disinfectants
    disinfectant log, 60
    Environmental Protection Agency (EPA)-
        approved, 56
    proper use of, 56
    tips and safety for, 59, 59f
Disorders and diseases of eye area
    allergic conjunctivitis, 37, 37f
    allergy vs. sensitivity
        patch tests, 44
        sensitization, 42
        skin reactions, reasons for, 42–43
    blepharitis, 37, 37f
    chalazion, 38, 38f
    conjunctivitis, 37, 37f
    contact dermatitis
        allergic, 39
        irritant, 39, 39f
    demodex, 38, 38f
    dry eye syndrome, 39
    eyelid and lash disorders, 40t
    ocular herpes, 40, 40f
    ocular rosacea, 38, 38f
    seborrheic dermatitis, 40, 40f
    stye, 38, 38f
    workbook assessment, 41, 45–46
Disposable implements. See Single-use
    implements

Index

Downturned eyes, 23t
Dramatic/maximum lashes, 117
Dry eye syndrome, 39
Dyes, as allergen, 43

E

Ectropion, 40t
Egyptians
    kohl makeup, creating, 5, 5f
    malachite, use of, 5, 5f
Elizabethan Era
    dyes for eyebrows/eyelashes, 6, 6f
Emergency eye cleansing protocol, 126
Employee injury, 82–83
Entropion, 40t
Equipment, disinfection of, 57
Equipment, for eyelash/eyebrow services
    adjustable light or magnifying light glasses, 96
    autoclave, 96
    hydraulic table, 96
    lash cart/trolley, 96
    technician's chair, 96
    trash container, 96
Ethics. *See also* Eyelash business development
    defined, 208
    ethical communication, 209
    professional, 209
Ethyl-Cyanoacrylate, 87
Exposure incidents
    blood exposure, 64
    eyewash stations, 65
    personal protective equipment, 65
    standard precautions, 64
External hordeolum, 38
Eye
    anatomy of, 19, 19f
    shapes, 23, 23t
    spacing on face, 25–27
        facial shapes, 26t
        workbook assessment, 28–29
Eyebrow lamination. *See also* Chemical services
    aftercare, 180–181
    contraindications, 180
    procedure, 180, 193–195
    troubleshooting, 181, 181f
Eyebrows
    anatomy of, 20, 20f
    functions of, 20
    sections of, 20, 20f
Eyebrow tinting, 105
    about, 186, 186f
    contraindications, 187
    procedure for, 199–200
    troubleshooting, 187

Eye irritations, 124
Eyelash business development, 204–223
    ethics
        defined, 208
        ethical communication, 209
        professional, 209
    marketing, 216
        branding, 217
        business cards, 218
        ideas, 219, 219f
        innovation in, 217, 217f
        social media, 218
        viral marketing, 218
    overview, 204
    pricing services, 213, 213f
    product line
        aftercare, 211
    professional image
        personal grooming, 205–206
        personal hygiene, 206
        professional attitude, 206–207, 206f
    retailing, 215
    social media
        content of post, 222
        time to post, 221
        use of, 221, 221f
    workbook assessment, 207–208, 210–211, 212–213, 214–215, 216, 220–221, 222–223
Eyelash cleanser, 103
Eyelash cleansing brushes, 95
Eyelash curler, invented by William Mcdonell, 7t
Eyelashes
    anatomy of, 20
    functions of, 20
    hair growth
        anagen stage, 30
        catagen stage, 30
        telogen stage, 30
        workbook assessment, 31–3
    tints, 105
Eyelash extension
    curl, 100, 100t
    diameter and length, 100–101, 100f
    eyelash industry, overview of, 4, 12
    eyelash technicians, 4, 9, 12
    faux mink lashes, 99
    history of
        early beginnings, 5–7, 7t
        modern eyelash extensions, 7
    mink lashes, 99
    products, 104
    scope of practice and laws, 9
    silk lashes, 99
    synthetic lashes, 99
    workbook assessment, 8, 10–11, 13–14

Index

Eyelash extension adhesive
　carbon black, 88
　cyanoacrylate, 87
　drying vs. curing, 88, 88f
　formaldehyde, 88
　humidity and temperature, 89
　hydroquinone, 88
　polymethyl methacrylate, 88
　storage, 89
Eyelash extension application
　classic eyelash application, 132, 132f
　　application variation, 132
　　lash extension placement, 132
　　procedure for, 132, 153–155
　client aftercare, 142–143, 143f
　client consultation
　　consultation form, 114, 114f–115f
　　preparing client for, 113
　contraindications, 124
　eyelash refill, 137, 137f
　　procedure for, 159–160
　lashes, types of, 118
　lash map, 120–121, 120f, 121f
　overview, 112
　preparation for extensions, 126–128
　　practising, 128, 128f
　proper extension, choice of, 117, 117f
　removal procedure, 140, 140f, 161–163
　temporary eyelash application
　　procedure for, 147–152
　　removing, 131
　　types of, 130, 130f
　troubleshooting, 144–145
　volume eyelash applications
　　characteristics, 135, 135f
　　lash fan creation, 136, 136f
　　procedure for, 156–158
　workbook assessment, 116, 118–119, 122–123,
　　125–126, 128–129, 133–134, 137,
　　138–139, 141–142, 143–144, 145–146
Eyelash industry
　career development in, 12
　growth of, 12
　lash salon owners, 12
　overview of, 12
Eyelash lifting. *See also* Chemical services
　aftercare, 177
　consultation, 176, 176f
　contraindications, 177
　and lamination product, 104–105, 105f
　other lash procedures, 177
　patch tests for, 44
　preparation, health, and safety, 177
　procedure for, 189–192
　skin reactions from, 43
　troubleshooting, 177–178, 177f
Eyelash refill, 137, 137f
　procedure for, 159–160
Eyelash separation tool, 93
Eyelash technicians
　on anatomy/physiology, 9
　on business of eyelashes, 204
　on client safety and infection control, 50
　demand of, 12
　on disorders, diseases, and allergies of eye, 36
　earnings of, 12
　on eye/eyelash anatomy, 18
　on eyelash and eyebrow chemical services, 170
　on eyelash extension application, 112
　on eyelash extension tools, products and
　　ingredients, 86
　goal of, 4
　licensing, certification, and governing laws, 9
　medical professional/licensed cosmetologist, 9
　objective and priority of, 9
　scope of practice, 9
　studying disorders/diseases/allergies of eye, 36
　training of, 9
　understanding of eyelash extension history, 4
Eyelash tinting. *See also* Chemical services
　aftercare, 184
　contraindications, 183
　preparation, health, and safety, 184
　procedure for, 183, 183f, 196–198
　troubleshooting, 184
Eyelid and lash disorders, 40t
Eyelids
　anatomy of, 19, 19f
　glands of, 19f
　hairs sewn onto, 6
　shapes of, 23, 23t
Eye pads, 94
　patch tests, 44
　skin reactions from, 42
Eyewash stations, 65

F

Face, eye spacing on, 25–27
Facial shapes, 26t
Faux mink lashes, 99
Feminine lashes, 117
Fire-fighting measures, 62
First-aid measures, 62
Formaldehyde, 88
Fragrances, as allergen, 42
Free consultations, 219

Index

G
Galena, black mineral, 5, 5f
Gel chemical remover, 140f
Gel in eye pads, allergic, 42
Gift certificates, 219
Glands of Zeis, 19
Glaucoma, 124
Gloves, 65, 65f
Glue rings, 95
Granuloma, 38

H
Hand sanitizers, waterless, 54
Hand washing, 53, 69–70
    waterless hand sanitizers, 54
Heart face shape, 26t
History of eyelash extension
    early beginnings, 5–7, 7t
    modern period, 7
Hooded eyes, 23t
Hordeolum, 38
Humidity and temperature, 89
Hydraulic table, 96
Hydroquinone, 88
Hygiene standard, 51

I
Implements
    defined, 92
    multiuse
        eyelash separation tool, 93
        jade stone or crystal, 93
        lash tile or lash palette, 93, 93f
        mini fan/bulb syringe, 94
        mirror, 94
        silicone eyelash lifting shields and rods, 94, 94f
        trimming scissors, 93
        tweezers, 92–93
    single-use, 94–95, 94f, 95f
Individual lashes, 130
Infection control basics, 51
Interdental brushes, 95, 95f
Internal hordeolum, 38
Irritant contact dermatitis, 39, 39f

J
Jade stone or crystal, 93

K
Kohl makeup
    use in Egypt, 5, 5f
Kohl tube and stick, 5f

L
Lacrimal gland, 19
Lamination, eyebrow
    skin reactions from, 43
Lash. *See also* Eyelashes
    cart/trolley, 96
    cleanser, 143f
    extension placement, 132
Lashes, types of, 118
Lash fans
    creation of, 136, 136f
    perfect, 135f
    use in volume eyelash applications, 135
Lash map
    cat-eye lash map, 121, 121f
    defined, 120
    open-eye lash map, 120, 120f
    suitable for client, 121
    textured lash map, 121, 121f
Lash tile or lash palette, 93, 93f
Latex adhesive, 43
Latex gloves, 65
Lifting, eyelash. *See also* Eyelash lifting
    and lamination product, 104–105, 105f
    patch tests for, 44
    skin reactions from, 43
Lint-free applicators, 95
Local corporations, 219

M
Madarosis, 40t
Malachite, use of, 5, 5f
Manual removal, 140
Marketing, 216. *See also* Eyelash business development
    branding, 217
    business cards, 218
    ideas, 219, 219f
    innovation in, 217, 217f
    social media, 218
    viral marketing, 218
Mascara
    brushes for, 94
    invented by Eugene Rimmel, 6
    in Victorian Era, 6

Index

Masks, 65
Mcdonell, William, 7t
Medical-grade adhesive, 7
Medical tape, 94
Meibomian glands, 19
Methoxy-Cyanoacrylate, 87
Methyl-Cyanoacrylate, 87
Micro swabs, 94, 94f
Middle age women
 removing hair from eyebrows/eyelashes, 6, 6f
Mink lashes, 99
Modern eyelash extensions, 7
Monolid eyes, 23t
Multiuse implements
 eyelash separation tool, 93
 jade stone or crystal, 93
 lash tile or lash palette, 93, 93f
 mini fan/bulb syringe, 94
 mirror, 94
 silicone eyelash lifting shields and rods, 94, 94f
 trimming scissors, 93
 tweezers, 92-93
Multiuse products, 58
Mutagen, 62

N
Nano mister, 94
Natural eyelash extension, 117, 117f
Nebulizer, 94
Nefertiti with kohl-lined eyes, 5f
Nessler, Karl, 7t
Nitrile gloves, 65, 94

O
Oblong face shape, 26t
Occupational Safety and Health Administration (OSHA) Hazard Communication Standard, 60
Ocular herpes, 40, 40f
Ocular rosacea, 38, 38f
Open-eye lash map, 120, 120f
Oval face shape, 26t
Overprocessing of lashes, 43

P
Palpebral conjunctiva, 19
Patch tests
 for adhesive, 44, 44f
 adverse reaction, handling, 44
 for eye pads, 44
 for lifting, 44
 for tape, 44
 for tinting, 44
Permanent eyelash lifting. See Eyelash lifting
Perming. See Eyelash lifting
Personal grooming, 205-206
Personal habits, 51
Personal hygiene, 206
Personal protective equipment (PPE), 65
Petroleum-based gloves, 65
Pinkeye. See Conjunctivitis
Pliny the Elder, 5
Polymerization, 88
Polymethyl methacrylate (PMMA), 88
Pricing services, 213, 213f
Product line, 211
Professional attitude, 206-207, 206f
Professional dress, 205
Professional ethics, 209
Professional image
 personal grooming, 205-206
 personal hygiene, 206
 professional attitude, 206-207, 206f
Prominent (protruding), 25t
Public relations events, 219

Q
Queen Elizabeth I, 6f
Queen Victoria, 6f

R
Referral and recommendation, 218
Retailing, 215
Rimmel, Eugene (Victoria's perfumer)
 creating mascara, 6, 6f
Romans
 use of kohl for eyelash enhancement, 5, 5f
 on women's lashes, 5, 5f
Round eyes, 23t
Round face shape, 26t
Round tweezers, 92

S
Safety data sheet (SDS), 60-62, 60f, 61f
 vocabulary, 62
Sclera, 19
Sebaceous glands, 19
Seborrheic dermatitis, 40, 40f

Index

Sensitization, 42
Service products and ingredients
    eyelash and eyebrow tints, 105
    eyelash cleanser, 103
    eyelash extension products, 104
    lifting and lamination product, 104–105, 105f
Shapes
    of eye and eyelid, 23, 23t
    workbook assessment, 24–25
Silicone eyelash lifting shields and rods, 94, 94f
Silk lashes, 99
Single-use implements, 94–95, 95f
    adhesive stickers, 95
    client headbands, 94
    cotton pads, 95
    eyelash cleansing brushes, 95
    eye pads, 94
    glue rings, 95
    glue rings and glue cups, 95
    interdental brushes, 95, 95f
    lint-free applicators, 95
    mascara brushes, 94
    medical tape, 94
    micro swabs, 94, 94f
    nitrile gloves, 94
    Y combs, 95, 95f
Single-use items, handling of, 58
Skin reactions, reasons
    adhesives
        dyes, 43
        latex, 43
    eyebrow lamination, 43
    eyelash and eyebrow tinting, 43
    eyelash application too close to skin, 43
    eyelash lifting, 43
    eye pads, 42
    improper isolation, 43
    symptoms, 42
    tapes, 42
Slant tweezers, 92
Social media. See also Eyelash business development
    content of post, 222
    influence on eyelash products, 7
    and marketing, 218
    time to post, 221
    use of, 221, 221f
Soft skills, 206
South Korea
    semi-permanent eyelash extensions, 7
Square face shape, 26t
Staphylococcus
    causing blepharitis, 37, 37f
Sterilizers, 57, 57f
Stoka, Katy, 7
Straight tweezers, 92
Strip lashes, 130, 130f
Stye, 38, 38f
Synthetic black lashes, 117
Synthetic lash, 99

T

Tape
    patch tests for, 44
    skin reactions from, 42
Taping technique, 127, 127f
Taylor, Anna, 7t
Tear films, 19
Technician's chair, 96
Telogen stage, eyelash hair growth, 30
Temporary eyelash adhesive, 90, 90f
Temporary eyelash application
    cluster lashes, 130, 150–152
    individual lashes, 130
    procedure for, 147–152
    removing, 131
    strip lashes, 130, 130f
Textured lash map, 121, 121f
Time management, 207
Tinting, eyelash and eyebrow
    patch tests for, 44
    skin reactions from, 43
Tools, products and ingredients, 86–107
    adhesives
        eyelash extension adhesive, 87–89, 88f
        temporary eyelash adhesive, 90, 90f
    equipment, 96–98
    eyelash extension curl, 100, 100t
    eyelash extension diameter and length, 100–101, 100f
    eyelash extensions
        types of, 99
    implements
        multiuse, 92–94, 93f, 94f
        single-use, 94–95, 94f, 95f
    overview, 86
    service products and ingredients
        eyelash and eyebrow tints, 105
        eyelash cleanser, 103
        eyelash extension products, 104
        lifting and lamination product, 104–105, 105f
    workbook assessment, 91, 97, 101–102, 106–107

Trash container, 96
Triangle face shape, 26t
Trichiasis, 40t
Trimming scissors, 93
Tweezers, 92–93
Twentieth century
    beauty industry expansion in, 6
    eyelash enhancement inventions, 7t

U
United States
    synthetic, single eyelash extensions, 7
Upturned eyes, 23t

V
Victorian Era
    cosmetics, use of, 6, 6f
    mascara, development of, 6, 6f
Viral marketing, 218
Volume eyelash applications
    characteristics, 135, 135f
    lash fan creation, 136, 136f
    procedure for, 156–158
Volume lashes, 118
Volunteer, 219

W
Waterless hand sanitizers, 54
Wide set eyes, 25t

Notes

Notes

Notes

Notes